The Wisdom of t

Finding Personal Truth
in the
too-much-information age

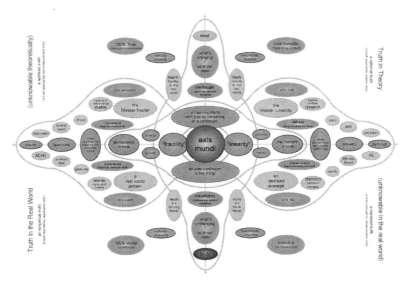

Book I: Solving the
Mind-Body Mystery

Steven Paglierani

published by

The Emergence Alliance™
Nanuet, New York

Emergence Alliance Publishing
55 Old Nyack Tpke., Ste 608
Nanuet, NY 10954

SAN 859-5380

http://StevenPaglierani.com (Musings, videos, announcements, and such. You can also download **full color drawings** from all my books here.)
http://theEmergenceSite.com (This site contains the twenty plus years of discoveries which led to this book. And while I've since refined many of my terms and ideas, some may find this earlier work of interest.
https://Vimeo.com/theScienceOfDiscovery (or search Vimeo for my name)
Here you'll find recent videos explaining many of my discoveries.

Paglierani, Steven. T., 1946-
    Solving the Mind-Body Mystery
    Book I in the Finding Personal Truth series

Cover Author-Photo Credit: Alistair Burke

Includes bibliographical references.

ISBN 978-0-9844895-3-4 (soft cover)
ISBN 978-0-9844895-6-5 (ebook)
ISBN 978-0-9844895-0-3 (hard cover, jacket)

1. Mind Body Mystery 2. Mind First, Body First 3. What is a fact?
4. Finding Personal Truth 1. title

242 pages. 92,000 words.

PHI015000   PHILOSOPHY / Mind & Body
PSY023000   PSYCHOLOGY / Personality
SCI075000   SCIENCE / Philosophy & Social Aspects

Library of Congress Control Number: 2010935644

Printing Number
    22 21 20 19 18   10 9 8 7 6 5 4 3 2

Dedication

To my parents, Aldo and Teresa, for teaching me to love learning. And to my fifth grade teacher. I hope, with this book, that I've finally vindicated myself. And that my original ideas will suffice.

Preface to the Paperback Version of Book I: January, 2018

Recently, I began to write what I hope will become the 4th book in this series. At this point, it's been close to eight years since I published Book I. In all this time, I've not found it in me to release paperback versions. And in part, I've simply been too busy making new discoveries to find the time.

I've also had the best group of formal students I've ever had. In addition, I've begun to develop physical models which allow people to personally interact with my ideas. Mainly though, I've felt discouraged, as most people find my books too hard to read. Indeed, one man recently complained, it takes him twenty minutes to read a single page. On a good day. Even then, he said, he often feels like throwing the book at a wall.

He then added, if I'd wanted people to understand my books, I'd have made them easier to read. Logically, he's right. In truth though, I've known about this problem for some time now. Indeed, two summers ago, when I published the third book in this series, I felt certain I'd done better. But recently, one of my brightest students told me, Book III is the hardest of all.

The thing is, when I parse my books through reading difficulty software, it tells me they are written at a fifth grade level. So what's going on here?

Logical Answers Which End (or avoid) Suffering

Just prior to publishing the third book, I stumbled onto what at first seemed to be just another piece of the puzzle. It involves something I've longed to understand: how a child's developing mind decides what to pay attention to and retain. In part, this learning resembles how we come to feel alert in dark rooms and high places. But in this case, our minds create a set of filters through which all life experiences must pass.

Experiences which pass through these filters get seen as important. They alone get processed and retained. Unfortunately, much of what's in my books doesn't pass through these filters. So even when people do momentarily comprehend what I write, moments later they remember nothing.

Where do these filters come from? They likely result from a common, early childhood event—a day wherein mommy or daddy suddenly got upset then yelled, "why did you do that?" If this kind of event startles you—even once—these filters get installed. Afterwards whole categories of life experience become hard to process or retain.

What makes this happen? These parents are demanding *logical* explanations. Children cannot understand logic until they can tell time. Most of us learn to tell time roughly at around age seven. So when a parent threatens to punish a three-year-old if they cannot logically explain why something happened, they panic. This panic then biases their minds. From then on, they know, "To avoid punishment, I must always have answers." The thing is, they're not old enough to use logic to find answers. So this makes them start doing the next best thing—they learn to fabricate answers. And herein lies the problem with reading my books.

Books filled with *"logical answers* to avoid *suffering"* become best sellers—even if most of what's in these books is totally fabricated nonsense. But books which focus mainly on the nature of things—and not on logical answers to suffering—are hard to read. Even if what's in them is true.

Why *suffering?* Parents do not suddenly scream, "why did you do that?" when good things happen.

Why *answers?* "Why did you do that?" is a demand for an answer.

Why *logic?* There are just two kinds of "why" questions—*natural* and *logical.*

Natural why questions request *descriptions* of natural processes. And the form these answers most often take is, "this, then this, *then* this."

Logical why questions request *logical explanations* for natural processes. And the form these answers most often take is, "this, then this, *therefore* this."

No coincidence, the three authorities we turn to most voice their work in the second manner. Here, science focuses on answering questions about how things do and don't work. Medicine focuses on finding and fixing what's wrong; on ending suffering. And psychology focuses on logically explaining who we are and why we suffer. And in truth, this should not be a surprise.

Scientists, doctors, and psychologists were once children too.

So again, why are my books hard to read? Because the human mind is biased to pay attention to—and retain—only *logical answers which end (or avoid) suffering.* My books don't focus on suffering They describe the nature of us and our world. This means your mind will likely filter out most of the content in this book. And the little that does make it through will get quickly forgotten.

So Can You Retain What You Read Here?

So here's the big question—can you retain what you read in this book? If you slow down, then focus on three things, you can improve your chances.

One, you'll need to focus on discovering *new lines of questioning*, rather than on finding answers. Two, you'll need to focus on finding *what's right about this book,* rather than what's wrong. And three (and hardest of all), you'll need to focus on *learning to observe the nature of things*, rather than on finding logical explanations for things. Especially the nature of this book's four main words: facts, stories, ideas, and feelings.

Is this a lot to ask from a reader? Admittedly, it is. But as you've no doubt found out, finding personal truth is never easy. Don't give up.

A Few Pointers Which I Hope Will Help the Reader

At some point, a writer has to concede, he or she will make no more revisions. But releasing a new edition can sometimes cause an author to revisit this concession. In my case, for a while, I felt sorely tempted to refine much of this book. In the end, common sense prevailed, and I chose to limit these revisions to minor changes and typos.

The thing is, this left me with a strong desire to help folks who may find reading this book hard. The following are a few suggestions which, eight years later, may help.

[1] Skip to Chapter Four, Then Read the Appendix

To begin with, I'd advise that you skip ahead to Chapter Four. And since my subheads anchor my ideas, don't skip over them—read them slowly. Next slowly read through the examples in the appendix, each of which changed a life. If you then feel curious, try reading the book from the beginning.

Why this order? Because Chapter Four should have come first. In it, I introduce what I now see as one of my most important discoveries. The discovery? That like handedness, there are only two possible mind body orientations. And each orientation has an up side and a down.

Mind first people sense life events first through their minds, as words. They think quickly on their feet. So the world sees them as smart. But they tend to overlook sensory cues, making them base decisions—like what and how much to eat—not on taste or fullness, but on logic and ideas. Great for publishers of diet books. Not so great if you're trying to lose weight.

Body first people—on the other hand—sense life events first through their bodies, as sensations. This means, most times, they process words as sensations, not as ideas. In general, they tend to use fewer words, and speak slower and less often. And this lack of words—and tendency to find their words slowly, gets seen as evidence for all manner of personal problems. Not caring. A lack of focus which requires medical interventions. Not wanting to talk things out.

Admittedly, body first people do act this way at times. Wouldn't you if the world kept telling you this is who and what you are? But do these tendencies mean they're less intelligent or that they don't care? Absolutely not. So what do they mean? Read chapter four.

[2] Create a Set of Wise Men's Cards and Use Them

Imagine using only words to describe a cumulus cloud to someone who has never seen one? Similarly, imagine trying to describe a candle flame with just words to a person born blind? These same limitations apply to your mind—you cannot learn from words alone.

This includes the words in this book.

On the other hand, in the first half of Book III, I introduce you to a new way to learn from words. It's called, "logical geometry," because you use it to arrange groups of words into geometric patterns. It turns out, it's these patterns which reveal the true meanings of words—and in the case of the wise men's card game, the biases in the way you seek truth.

What kinds of biases? How much or how little your mind uses time, place, and the mind's four domains—facts, stories, ideas, and feelings. Too few feelings? Too many facts. Well, you get the idea. To gain from this game though, you must do more than read. You must actually play.

[3] Create a List of Questions as You Read

In Book III, I also posit that a legitimate scientific method should focus not on answers but rather, on questions—that this shift in focus significantly increases one's chances for making discoveries. The point of course is, if you think you know an answer, then your mind closes and you stop looking. And closed minds do not make discoveries.

With this in mind, I'd like to offer you a few questions which may help to open and focus your mind. Do try to add to this list as you read.

- Does our experience of having a mind result entirely from our having a body? Is the mind just neurons firing? Do "neurons firing" equate to consciousness? If so, where's the evidence?
- According to this book, we can have ideas about feelings and we can have feelings about ideas. But we cannot have both at the same time. Can this be true? If so, is this why we hate being asked, "So how did that make you feel?"?
- This book claims our *mental* experience of a separate mind and body is rooted in our sense of time. Specifically, it claims the speed at which we process life determines *where* we process our experiences—in our minds or bodies. It further claims we each default to processing life either in the mind or the body—moreover, that the place we default to determines our sense of how smart we are. Can these things be true?
- This book also claims, our *physical* sense that the mind and body are separate is rooted in physiology. Specifically, it claims, we literally have two functioning, physical "brains"; the cranial and the enteric. Is there scientific proof for this? If so, why do scientists continue to ignore and overlook this?

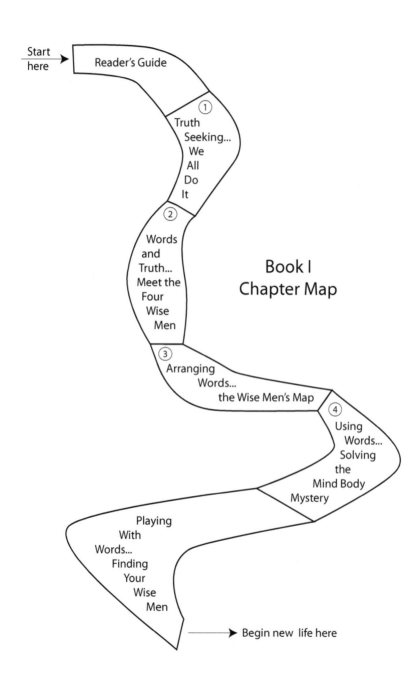

Start here

Reader's Guide

① Truth Seeking... We All Do It

② Words and Truth... Meet the Four Wise Men

③ Arranging Words... the Wise Men's Map

④ Using Words... Solving the Mind Body Mystery

Book I
Chapter Map

Playing With Words... Finding Your Wise Men

Begin new life here

Table of Contents

Chapter 2

Words and Truth—Meet the Four Wise Men   41

Chapter 3

Arranging Words—The Wise Men's Map   109

Chapter 4

Using Words—Solving the Mind Body Mystery 143

Appendix

Introduction

Reader's Guide to a Very Long Book

My Search For An Original Idea

If I was to tell you I began writing this book in fifth grade, you would probably think me mad. And you'd be right. I'm now in my sixties. How much could I even remember from fifth grade? In truth though, all things do begin somewhere. And this book did begin in fifth grade, when, for some now obscure reason, the teacher began the day by telling us that in all likelihood, no one in the class would ever have an original idea.

The thing is, I do have a kind of madness. I have Asperger's. So my reaction to her proclamation wasn't normal to say the least. To wit, from that morning on, her words so haunted me that I felt obligated to prove her wrong. Or die trying.

Looking back, my obsession almost did kill me. Many, many times. Then in August 1996, just four months shy of my fiftieth birthday, I had my first original idea. While meditating on a small mountain near my home, I realized that underlying every personal struggle is the same seemingly innocuous event—being startled. In other words, it's not traumas, symptoms, dysfunction, or mistakes which make our lives hard. It's startles. That's it. Just startles.

Does my claim about startles seem crazy? If so, don't be concerned. To be honest, back then, I had no idea what this realization meant, let alone that it would change the lives of so many people. Ironically, today, on days when I'm feeling more grandiose than I normally do, I imagine this moment as being similar to Descartes' grand realization; that thinking proves we exist. Ultimately, his certainty about the nature of thinking led to all his accomplishments. So my certainty about the nature of startles has led to mine.

Indeed, one month later, in September 1996, I had my second original idea. In a flash of insight, I realized that the only way to actually heal a wound is to have an aha while reliving the startle. And because this idea—that epiphanies heal wounds—is the complementary opposite to the first, I now had what I've come to call, a "personal truth."

Why write a book on how to find personal truth? For one thing, because we live in the "too-much-information" age. We need a way to tell nonsense from truth. For another, because my discovery—that startles burn out parts of our minds—means we are all prone to miscalculations in our search for truth, expert and amateur alike.

In addition, as a therapist, I've been haunted by how inexact talk therapy is. What we are taught about the mind and body feels vacuous and flawed. Finally, I have my personal reasons. As I've mentioned, I have Asperger's. Thus over the course of my life, I have, at one time or another, inadvertently offended almost every person I have ever come in contact with and never understood why.

For all these reasons and more, finding personal truth became my obsession. And in the years following those two insights, I tried in vain to share what I'd discovered. In the end, I found I had grossly misunderstood the nature of these discoveries. And my own inability to teach them. This led me to do what any madman who was bad at teaching would do. I started a school. And while at first, most of my students ended up leaving with middle fingers raised and cursing me as they exited, gradually, a few began to see me as sincere.

Then in June 2008, I had the aha that led to this series of books. While struggling to find a way to introduce my ideas to a new student, I accidentally stumbled onto what I now know to be a map of the human mind. Sounds like more craziness, doesn't it? A map of the human mind. Weeks later though, when I introduced this map to my students, I found myself talking about my discoveries in language that made my years of failure melt away.

This is how the four wise men were born. The map naturally delineates the mind into four interrelated parts. And because I love telling stories, I made these four divisions the mythical realms of four wise men and the truths that exist within these realms their four wisdoms.

Since then, I have come to love these four old curmudgeons and their wisdoms. And while I now see their bickering as the main impediment to knowing yourself, I also see their struggles as embodying the amazing courage and resilience of the human soul seeking truth.

As for why you are now facing a three volume work of epic proportions rather than a nice, slim, in-ten-easy-lessons book on finding personal truth, it's simple. These two ideas—that startles wound our minds and bodies, and that epiphanies heal these wounds—underlie every aspect of your personality. Including your consciousness. And while I realize how this must sound—boastful at the very least, and totally absurd at worst—perhaps peering into the mind of a madman might just be incentive enough for you to read on.

As for the concept behind these books, it's simple. One of my heroes, René Descartes, once wrote a book about how to discover truth. And while he didn't exactly call his method a way to find "personal" truth, he begins his book by telling his readers, "this is how I found truth. It might work for you." Thus it's clear he intended this.

In this way, my books are but an echo of Descartes'. And while the centuries have turned him into one of the most misunderstood geniuses of all time, his idea—that we each must find our own truth—is perhaps the most important original idea of all.

These books are about how I found my personal truth. I hope, with all my heart, that they enable you to do the same.

What Makes Something an Original Idea?

In theory, there was a first human being, and this person had the original ideas from which all others came. Including mine. However, crediting this faceless predecessor for my discoveries doesn't seem quite right. At the same time, without the myriad original ideas my heroes have instilled in me, I might as well have been born a brainless slug. Thus somewhere inbetween giving no credit and all the credit lies the truth.

What exactly am I offering credit for? To tell you, I need to define what I mean by an "original" idea. An original idea is something which is so obviously true that we find it hard to believe no one has said it before. At the same time, in hindsight, we can see that the seeds for this idea have existed inside every human being ever born.

In this way, I see my discovering original ideas as similar to how world class chefs create new recipes from already existing ingredients. Only in my case, the ingredients have come largely from the ideas and exploits of my heroes, most of whom I've never met and never will. As well as from the many people who have inspired me over the years, quite a few of whom I have met, many, face to face.

To me then, these people deserve the credit for being the source of my books; the brave souls who posit original ideas, and the compassionate beings who inspire us to seek these ideas. Not coincidentally, my father fits into the former group and my mother into the latter, albeit, were either of them still alive I'm sure they'd both vehemently deny this.

Why my father?

His lifelong love of all things mechanical led him to become the perennial explorer of exploded drawings. Indeed, I have many early childhood memories wherein he is sitting in our living room, dark save one orange floor lamp, searching for just the right diagram which would allow him to repair a junk yard car engine, or rebuild a discarded lawn mower, or repair my mother's ten year old iron. And while I doubt my father, during his eighty-eight years, ever read a single shred of what most would consider literature, the fact that all his life he sought knowledge in books has in part made me who I am. My hunger for books never ceases. And my having to put what I've learned into diagrams very much reminds me of him.

As for having original ideas, when my father couldn't afford a tool, he would spend all day on Sundays inventing one. And when he came up with this tool, and he always did, he'd beam with the delight of an eighteen month old who had just learned to put the right blocks in the right holes. These discoveries were probably the reason my father remained vital all his life. And in a real sense, his two callings—learning and helping people—both derived from this.

My mother, on the other hand, was the person who taught me both to be excited about learning and to delight in someone else's learning. For instance, I recall coming home from school early in third grade and having her tell me I had misspelled the word "grammar." She then went in search of the family dictionary and returned, moments later, grinning. At which point, she delighted in telling me that she had been wrong and I had been right.

For some reason, this simple act of love has so affected me that, like my father's love of learning from books, her delight in my discoveries has stayed with me all my life. That my father, the original thinker, never went past sixth grade, and that my mother had schizophrenia all her adult life only makes these things more meaningful. And so poignant. And I often think of them when people tell me they have nothing to contribute to this world and never will. Bah!

Some Hints Which May Make Reading This Book Easier

The first and most important suggestion I could make regarding this book is—take nothing for granted. Question everything you think you know. And everything I say. This was Descartes' way and this is my way. And if you truly want to find your truth, this must become your way.

Second, for most people, reading means trying to ingest as much information as you can cram into your head. That's why we call studying for tests, "cramming." However, you're not going to get tested on what is in this book. So while cramming can work with books based on one or two main ideas, this book has far too many ideas, facts, and stories in it to ever fit into one head. Including into mine. This is why any attempt to retain all of what you read, or even to understand all of what you read, will only frustrate you and make you want to fling this book onto the nearest dung heap.

What will work, however, is to first label the parts, then see how these parts are arranged. And to understand what I mean by this, I need to tell you a story.

Recently my boiler stopped working on a very cold day. Figures, right? Fortunately, my best friend is a plumber. So I called him. However, as he began to tell me how to diagnose the problem, I started to freak out.

"Take the aquastat cover off and pull the relay lever."

(What the heck is an aquastat and how do I get the cover off? Relay lever? That silver thingy? It's pulled out as far as it will go. Is this the right lever? Will I break the stupid thing if I pull harder?)

"Can you hear the pilot burner?"

(The what? What kind of sound does a pilot burner make? I do hear something. But I don't know what it means. Am I going to blow up the whole house if I do it wrong? Can't you just come over and do it for me or at least, speak English?")

"If it's out, then pull the cover off the front of the boiler and look inside to see if you can see anything."

(Cover? Okay. I bent it a little, but it's off. Uh, oh. I need to take that silver plate off. Okay. Calm down and breathe. Two hex head screws? Shit. I need my nut driver set. Where the hell did I last see it? Crap, I don't remember where I put it. Okay. Here it is. Oh, my back. It's a darn tight fit in here. Whew. Finally. It's off. Now what am I looking for?)

Long story short, I got off the phone, then read the directions on the side of the boiler. I then proceeded to locate, and label with a magic marker, each and every thingy attached to the side of my boiler. Then, when my friend called back and when he started speaking in tongues again, I was ready. And to my surprise, this time, I understood everything he said.

My point? If you try to learn the ideas in these books just by reading the words, you'll learn very little and understand even less. Indeed, the more you try to reduce what you're reading to what you already know, the less you'll learn. However, if you make a habit of referring back to the diagrams, you'll do great. Better still, copy these diagrams into your own little notebook and make notes as you're reading. It worked for my father. It will work for you.

In addition, pay particular attention to the way I've used subheads throughout these books. These subheads divide what are admittedly complex topics into manageable sections. Moreover, if you suddenly notice words spilling aimlessly through your brain, go back to the last subhead you did understand and try to connect it to what you're having trouble with.

Finally, do write down the words or phrases that appear to be me speaking in tongues. Then do your best to let them be "unknowns" for now and just keep reading. And trust the process. If you give yourself time and use these hints, you will succeed. I promise.

Some Pointers Regarding the Content

All books have a theme. These books do too. Finding personal truth in the too-much-information age is the theme of these books.

Along with this though are a number of auxiliary themes, the main one being that to find this truth, you'll need a method.

In addition, there are assertions I make without which these books could not exist. That personality, like all living things, is fractal, not linear. That synchronicities do not prove all things happen for reasons. That our perception of time is what creates the mind body duality. That startles program blank spots into our minds that only epiphanies can heal.

In addition to these assertions, I make a number of assumptions as well. That all babies are born with an innate capacity, and desire, to find their own truth. That all people suffer injuries to this innate capability. That it takes more than logic and compassion to heal these injuries. That we all deserve this healing. And that only by doing this, can we get the lives we want.

Then there is the thing about how I write. People with Asperger's use words differently than normal people. Thus there are places in these books where you may feel annoyed by what appear to be redundancies and repetitions. In truth, I'm not repeating myself. I'm merely restating things in different words in order to add shades of meaning.

I also tend to redefine words a lot—facts, feelings, stories, and ideas being the main four. But there are literally hundreds of other words which I have felt the need to clarify or redefine. The Asperger's thing again. In chapter two, I address this need, and hopefully this will suffice.

Why tell you this? Because there will be times wherein you'll find yourself getting lost. Know that when this happens, it's probably not you. Rather it's likely you've been thrown off by a word or phrase for which you already have a meaning but which I have felt the need to refine. Here, a little patience will go a long way. This, and remembering what I've mentioned about how folks with Asperger's use words.

Finally, we come to the strange diagrams you'll find strewn amongst the pages. In these drawings, I marry classical geometry to aspects of fractal science. By doing this, complex truths transform into recognizable geometric shapes and shades of grey. Thus if you pay particular attention to these drawings, your mind and body will absorb far more than my words could ever communicate.

Of course, in order to access these truths, you'll need to relax and let them seep into your mind. In this way, these drawings resemble the magic eye drawings from a few decades back, you know, the ones you must relax to see. Then again, since the truth you seek will often be hiding in plain sight, right in front of you, this ability—to allow things to seep into your mind—will be an essential skill for you as a truth seeker. So again, be patient. And if you do your best to cultivate this skill, you will succeed.

How I've Organized the Chapters

Like many people I know, I hate being told what is and isn't true. No surprise then that I go to great lengths not to impose my truths on others. This said, it might be helpful to share my thoughts as to why I've structured the chapters as I have. And why the subtitle of this book refers to it as *Book I*. How many books are there?

In all, there will be three books, all titled, **Finding Personal Truth in the too-much-information age.** This book is **Book I: Solving the Mind-Body Mystery.** The next book will be **Book II: Unraveling Human Nature.** And the third book will be **Book III: Solving the Mysteries of the Universe.**

Know I had originally hoped to publish all three books under one cover. However, facing an 800 page tome can discourage even the most adventurous reader. Not to mention the cost.

At the same time, these three books are still really one long book. Thus I've opted to retain the original, single-book, chapter and page numbering scheme. And while you're welcome to read these books in any order you like, it's best to treat Book I as the beginner's course, Book II as the intermediate course, and Book III as the advanced course.

Book I: Solving the Mind-Body Mystery

As for what's in these books, let's start with the current book, Book I: Solving the Mind-Body Mystery. In it, you'll find chapters one through four, along with instructions for playing the wise men's game. What's it about?

As I've said, this book is the beginner's course. Thus, chapter one introduces you to the main ideas—that we all seek truth—that there are only four ways in which human beings seek truth—that in order to find your "personal" truth, you must have access to all four—and that a map of your mind, and a method for using this map, can allow you to combine all four in a way which gives you access to your own wisdom.

Why focus on a map and a method, rather than on telling you "the" truth? For one thing, because no matter what people tell you, there is no "one-size-fits-all" truth. For another, because even if there was, no amount of books could hold it all.

Mainly I do this though because, while I believe there are no inherently stupid people, a lot of us act stupid, by blindly accepting other people's truths rather than seeking our own.

At the same time, even the smartest people fall prey to self doubt at times. I surely do. Thus having the map and a method for using it can bolster your confidence and keep you on track.

So where is this map? Before I can tell you, I first need to introduce you to the four map makers. You'll meet them in chapter two. I'll also introduce you to their four wisdoms—facts, stories, ideas, and feelings. Here, we'll look at how we must use words in order to find truth. But because words can deceive and mislead us, we must do more than understand them. We must learn to picture them. Literally.

Admittedly, this chapter is dense, so reading it may feel overwhelming at times. And yes, this is ironic, considering this book's title. At the same time, it's not as distasteful as a colonoscopy and it's a lot more interesting. Moreover, since this chapter lays the foundation for the entire series of books, if you take it seriously and go slow, you'll benefit greatly.

In chapter three, I'll begin to reveal the secrets of the map, including how the four wisdoms fit into it. Here, you'll learn things like how the mind and body each have their own way of looking for truth, and why theoretical truths don't translate well to the real world. Admittedly, some of this stuff can feel like you're wading through philosophical molasses—the "five aspects of truth" (duality, unity, simultaneity, sums, and emergent properties), the mysterious "Axis Mundi," and the origin of the Tao symbol, for instance. On the other hand, if you like esoterica, you're going to love this chapter. And even if you don't, reading this chapter may change your mind.

Why have I made you read all this? You'll find out in chapter four. Here, you'll use what you've learned so far to solve a major mystery—how the mind and body connect—the real truth. What could I possibly say that has not been said before? Again, it's not the ingredients. It's the way these ideas are put together. All I can say is, be prepared to be stunned by how obvious the answer turns out to be. And by how many mysteries this answer unravels. The word here is *fun*.

Finally, I'll introduce you to the wise men's game, a powerful method for uncovering the inner workings of people's minds. From it, you'll discover which wise men you favor, and which you ignore. You may even heal a few wounds, albeit, I can't promise that. But whatever the case, you'll be well prepared for the next leg of your journey—discovering what it means to be human—the real story.

Book II: Unraveling Human Nature
To begin with, as a book, Book II—the intermediate level book—is a bit strange. It only has two chapters, five and six. It also contains a series of personality tests, the likes of which the world has never seen. Including my claim that the results of these tests are one hundred percent certain.

What's in it for you?

In chapter five, you'll learn that to find personal truth, you need a personality theory—a collection of assumptions as to what makes people tick. And lest this sound like something you have no interest in, know we all have these theories, albeit, you may never have called your "how-people-tick" thoughts, a theory.

The trouble with most of these theories, of course, is how they add to your information overload. Amazingly, this personality theory is so precise that a single drawing holds all of human nature. Every detail. Every nuance.

How is this possible?

Unlike previous theories, this one is fractal. By this, I mean, it unfolds in self-similar layers, sort of like the proverbial onion, or like Russian nesting dolls. At the same time, because the same ten recognizable patterns repeat throughout, this theory is infinitely complex. Yet it's so simple, even young children grasp the basics. And while this boast may sound suspiciously similar to a late night infomercial for the perfect car wax, I mean this literally. Indeed, one seven-year-old boy whose mother I'm close to recently taught parts of this theory to his class. Unsolicited. At age seven. You'll find his story later on in this book.

Again, this chapter has a lot of information in it. We are, after all, defining what it means to be human. Know that in chapter six, you'll be rewarded for all this work, when I introduce you to something I call your *core personality*—the part of you which, from age four on, never changes.

Imagine knowing exactly what makes you, you? Personality tests based on the wise men's theory can reveal this and more. Things like why you fall in love with the people you fall in love with and how you pick your friends. They can even match teachers to students and people to their careers. As well as improve your parenting skills and all your relationships.

Finally, at the end of Book II, you'll find the actual tests. Know they're unlike any personality tests you're even taken. For one thing, they're tipping-point based, which is what makes them one hundred percent accurate. For another, they're brief, fun, and deeply revealing. At the same time, they're so provocative, they sometimes provoke epiphanies in people. So it's just possible, taking these tests may change your life. And heal a few wounds, besides.

Book III: Solving the Mysteries of the Universe

In Book III—the advanced book—we'll broaden our focus to include the whole Universe. Here, we'll explore the mathematical, scientific, and pragmatic proof behind Books I and II. In short chapters with lots of pictures no less. Topics will include a new geometry which combines shapes with words—a new algebra which unifies the hard sciences, like physics, with the soft sciences, like psychology—a new mathematics which can measure real-world things with one hundred percent accuracy—and a new psychotherapy which can pin-point wounds so well that it makes conventional talk therapy seem like stone-age brain surgery.

We'll begin with chapter seven, where you'll learn how to map truth. Amazingly, the whole trick lies in using the map to arrange your words. These "word-maps" make it easy to discern between other people's truths and your own. As well as enabling you to master a wide variety of things, from to-do lists and Tai Chi classes to meditation and career advancement.

Realize that to make these word-maps, you'll need to learn a bit of geometry. Six geometric patterns to be exact. Here, we're talking about the six geometries from which all truth derives. Know that anyone who masters these patterns will be able to discover original ideas. As well as being able to know for sure whether something is true. Indeed, these patterns are so powerful that, in a few cases, learning this geometry has increased the person's IQ. And while I can't promise this will happen to you, I can't rule it out either.

In chapter eight, you'll learn how to fine tune your truth seeking, by ruling out things you cannot know. Here we'll look at how uncertainty drives us to try to predict the future. This is the obsession which drives us to trust so-called experts, rather than trusting ourselves. Fortunately for us, there's a remedy for this obsession—something called, the "personal uncertainty principle," a theorem which defines the limits of what we can know. Moreover, when you know this theorem, it takes the pressure off you, because it allows you to let go of what can't be known.

In chapter nine, you'll learn how to create maps of everything that occurs in your mind. Here, we'll explore the four fractal patterns from which all human experience derives, the four recognizable shapes which lie hidden within the seemingly chaotic data of your mind. To do this, we'll combine Cartesian coordinates with an algebra so powerful that it's capable of revealing the essential nature of every aspect of human consciousness—from mania, addiction, and getting overwhelmed to depression, healing, and being born. From this, you gain the ability to visually describe seemingly nebulous experiences—like feelings and addictions—with shapes. Can you imagine? A shape for depression. A shape for boredom. A shape for cocaine addiction and falling in love.

In chapter ten, I'll teach you the secrets to finding and healing wounds, beginning with that it's information-overloads which cause your wounds. And enable you to heal. I'll also teach you some evidence-based methods which could improve all therapies, psychological and physical alike. For instance, did you know that *bracing for pain*—whether in your mind or body—proves you have a wound, while experiencing pleasant surprise *after bracing for pain* is the proof this wound has healed?

I'll also tell you some healing stories which demonstrate the basic techniques from Emergence Therapy, the first talk therapy to focus directly on wounds, rather than on symptoms, illogic, or painful events. Here, you'll learn things like how ordinary words can sometimes wound you, and why some types of violence don't wound you. As well as a rather controversial assertion—that being molested doesn't always result in sexual wounds.

Speaking of healing stories, in chapter eleven, you'll hear a few more. This time, we'll focus on relationships and love—romantic, and otherwise. Again, we'll look to solve a few mysteries, things like why most parents disagree about how best to discipline their children, and why parents connect differently to each of their children. We'll also look at why you can find someone who, in theory, is your perfect mate, yet feel no attraction.

In chapter twelve, we'll look at learning, starting with the four-step sequence I call "personal" learning. What is personal learning? Learning you can't get enough of. Learning you never forget. Learning you never tire of revisiting. Learning that makes you feel young. Sounds a little like falling in love, doesn't it?

We'll also look at what makes people hate learning, and why kids drop out of school. And what makes some teachers boring. And how to recapture your early-childhood curiosity.

Finally, in chapter thirteen, I'll introduce what could become the future of science, something I call, "constellated science." This method enables lay people to make discoveries even in technically complex fields of study. Here, we'll constellate what is known about three topics—sleep problems, weight loss, and a rare kind of deafness—in hopes we'll unearth a few previously unseen possibilities hidden within this data. And while we may fail to uncover any fully-baked new truths, I expect we'll at least come up with some interesting paths for future exploration. As well as piss off a few closed-minded scientists.

Sound like a lot to cover? Trust me, you have no idea.

A Few Last Thoughts Before You Begin Your Adventure

Although we haven't met, and while this may make you uncomfortable, I have to say something before you begin.

I believe in you.

I also believe you have it in you to find your truth, and to use this truth to leave this world a better place for your having been in it. This said, it's likely you'll never read another series of books like this for as long as you live. Book publishers don't normally publish books which contain so many ideas. I've literally attempted to explain the essence of everything we experience as human beings—a "theory of everything personal," so to speak. And while I knew I would never succeed, I've tried anyway.

Try anyway.

Steven Paglierani

Chapter 1

Truth Seeking . . . We All Do It

Are You A Truth Seeker?

Do you consider yourself a *truth seeker?* Most people never ask themselves this question. Despite this oversight, we each in our own way seek truth every day. Most of us do this more in the personal sense of the word *truth* than in the abstract philosopher's sense. This is the kind of truth this book will teach you to find; your *personal* truth.

On what do I base this claim? On that I've discovered something astonishing about the human mind—that you can use fractals to map the pathways through it. In other words, despite the seemingly infinite variety of things you can think, feel, say, and do, beneath this apparent infinity lie a finite set of non-linear patterns. Fractal patterns, to be exact.

Moreover, because all human minds—like all human bodies—are based on the same set of non-linear patterns, these fractal patterns hold the key to understanding everything about you. How you learn. Who you'll love. How to find and heal your wounds. These patterns reveal it all. Imagine what it would be like to know these patterns—the mysteries you could solve? You could make sense of your childhood—and see where your deepest feelings go. You could figure out what's been wrong in your relationships and how to have a happy life. Imagine?

The Original Wise Men's Map

© 2008 Steven Paglierani, The Center for Emergence

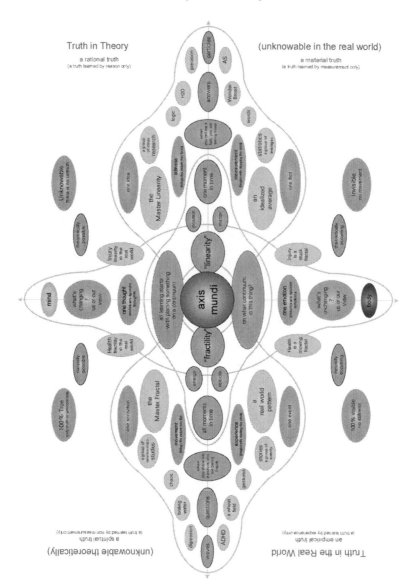

The problem is, while we all want these things, we mostly seek them with logic. But personal truths cannot be found with logic alone. Nor do they become visible just by looking into your heart. Indeed, under normal circumstances, many of these roads are just plain invisible. Except to those who know the secret to making them become visible—the special circumstances under which these pathways to personal truth appear.

In this book, we'll be referring to these special circumstances as "sitting with the four wise men"—four imaginary characters who together represent the four schools of thought we've been using to look or our truth. Rationalism. Materialism. Empiricism. Spiritualism. We all use these methods, even if these particular words seem unfamiliar to you.

Seen as the four wise men's wisdom, however, we become able to see the good in all four approaches. Together, they become the four roads which can lead us to our personal truth.

What are these roads like? The first are the super highways of ideas and logic. This is the way the *rationalist wise man* tells us to go. The second kind of roads are the city thoroughfares of facts and measurement. This is the way the *materialist wise man* tells us to go. Next come the small town roads of stories and experience. This is where the *empirical wise man* wants us go. Fourth come the dirt paths and overgrown fields of feelings and intuition. Here is where the *spiritual wise man* urges us to go.

Do these roads sound familiar? They should. You've been traveling on them all your life. Unfortunately, there are things about these roads no one has told you before. Take personal truth. Are you looking for it? Then you'll need to travel on all four kinds of roads. Like ingredients in a cake, you need all your ingredients in order to find your truth.

You also can't travel these roads separately, then add up what you find. Personal truth emerges only when you have what amounts to an aerial view. In a way then, trying to find personal truth is a lot like trying to find a destination on a conventional road map. To feel confident, you need more than just the location. You need to see the whole map.

Unfortunately, the wise men know that if you learn to see the whole map, you won't need them anymore. So they each tell you only their roads are safe and that the other wise men's roads are nothing but dead ends and dangerous curves.

Eventually, we all fall for this ruse and we come to trust one wise man above the rest. This causes us lose faith in ourselves. So we begin to seek our truth in others. In the end, we forget how to find our truth and mistake other peoples' truth for our own.

So much for finding our personal truth.

This then is the main problem with finding personal truth. Without realizing it, we each, in our own way, forget how to find it for ourselves. At the same time, because the world is hard on folks who don't know themselves, we feel vulnerable and stupid a lot. But to admit we've deferred to the truths of others can make us feel just as bad, sometimes worse.

How about when someone suggests you may have missed something? Do you ever overreact or feel compelled to explain yourself? What about when someone questions your decisions—do you ever get defensive? If so, don't feel embarrassed. We all get this way at times. Each time a wise man convinces us that he alone has the answers.

Later, when we realize we've been taken in, we feel sick at heart. And when we ask ourselves why we trusted him, we have little to say. Who are these wise men anyway, and how can they have so much power over us? Here, it's not hard to see. For some of us it's our doctor, and why not. Medical things are scary. For others it's a spiritual guide, something we all need from time to time. For some it's their professor, or therapist, or favorite author. After all, they're "authorities." And for others, it's their closest friend, the one who wants the best for them.

How does surrendering yourself to the minds of others affect your search for truth? To see, imagine you're facing a serious life decision, one which will change the course of your life. Something on the scale of having another child, or moving across the country, or changing your career. How would you go about making this kind of decision?

Ideally, now that I've told you that you need all four wise men, you'd consult them before making this decision. Okay. So imagine you're walking into the Hall of Wisdom. But the first thing you see is them arguing. Good grief! In fact, at one point, they're arguing so loudly that you consider leaving. But just as you're ready to shout, "hey, remember me!" they realize you're there. At which point, they quietly and contritely return to their seats, four rather impressive thrones arranged in a square, in the middle of which is a fifth chair. The chair reserved for you.

At this point, you start walking toward that fifth chair. But before you can sit, they make a request. With serious faces, they ask you to consider where you'll position your chair, as once you're in it, you can't move it. Okay, fine, you think. What's the big deal. I'm moving the chair. See. At which point, you realize they're all staring at you. Why? These dummies are waiting to see which of them your chair will face, in effect, deciding which of them is wisest and which one you'll turn your back on.

When faced with difficult decisions, this is how most of us behave. We blindly accept our trusted wise man's advice and ignore the advice of the rest. Or at times, we do consider what others have to say. But if their advice doesn't match our wise man, we dismiss it as stupid or flawed.

What about the fourth wise man, the one we turn our back on? What happens to his advice? Basically, we ignore it and act as if it wasn't even said. After all, who takes seriously the advice of a stupid person? No one I know. And this is our biggest mistake. As I said, to find personal truth, we need all four wise men. Thus, we need this wise man's advice most of all.

All this changes when you learn to see the map. We'll talk about how to do this in chapter two. We'll also discuss how not including all four wise men in our decisions leads to our prejudices and blind spots. We'll talk about this in all three books, but especially in Book III. I'll also be teaching you something you're sure to like, something I call, "the method." Here you'll learn a quick yet powerful way to use the map to find personal truth.

Along the way, I'll also share some of what my own searches for personal truth have led me to, including a pretty interesting and previously unknown explanation for how the mind and body connect (chapter four), as well as how this connection, or lack thereof, leads us to fight with those we love (Book III: chapter eleven) and struggle to learn new things (Book III: chapter twelve).

Of course, our main focus throughout this series of books will be on finding personal truth, beginning with defining what it is. You see, personal truth is not the kind of truth people normally seek. Most folks seek *the* truth. You know, the one and only, forever and always, ultimate, perfect truth. This makes the idea of a *personal* truth pretty hard to define, especially when so many folks argue about what makes something true.

So what is personal truth? It's simple, really. It's what emerges in you whenever you and all four wise men simultaneously agree on something. In other words, it's what you find when you consciously see your destination and the whole map together. Seeking this commonality between you and the four wise men—by seeing your destination and the whole map—is how you find personal truth. And the more you learn to do this, the better your life becomes.

Do You Really Need Help Finding Your Truth?

Okay. Yes. I know. I've put a lot out there, including some pretty arcane sounding stuff. *Fractal pathways through the mind? Sitting with the four wise men? The secret to finding your personal truth?* Sounds a lot like new-age nonsense, doesn't it? The thing to notice, though, is not whether you think I'm full of shit. Rather, it's how you're deciding if this book is for you. What's going through your head?

In truth, I haven't explained much. So if you're already trying to decide whether to keep reading, then ask yourself this. How often do you make decisions based on this little information? Frequently? All the time? Rarely? Once in a while? I bring this up because how you decide whether or not to read this book will have a lot in common with how you make all your personal decisions. Including that being intelligent in no way substitutes for having enough information.

This raises an interesting question. Do folks born with exceptional minds generally make better decisions? Not surprisingly, the answer depends a lot on how you define *intelligence*. You see, in general, the word *intelligence* refers to two things—[1] to our ability to picture things, and [2] to our ability to mentally recognize patterns in what we see. IQ tests literally test for these two things. And yes, being intelligent obviously factors into whether you'll find your personal truth. But when it comes to personal truth, it's far from the end all be all some would have us believe.

To see what I'm saying, consider the part intelligence plays in baking cakes. Yes, being intelligent means we can read a cake recipe. And comprehend the directions. But does it guarantee how this cake will taste? Of course not. No more than intelligence explains why we see roses as beautiful, or feel drawn to puppies and newborns. Or why your neighbor's oldest daughter, a certified genius, has been dating what appears to be a Neanderthal.

My point is, regardless of how smart you are, you will need more than intelligence to find your personal truth.

What if you see yourself as only average? Or less than average? Dumb even. Do dumb people have a harder time finding their personal truth? My take on this? I believe there are no inherently dumb people. There are only folks who act dumb, by deferring to the truths of others. How many people do this? Most people. Which is why so many of us struggle all our lives to know ourselves.

What makes a smart person smart then is that they won't do this. At least, not when it counts. Take my friends John and Jen. Recently they faced a grave personal decision—whether or not to have their deaf two year old son, Aidan, get cochlear implants. Not surprisingly, with several referrals in hand, they still felt insecure and uncertain as to which doctor to choose. Can you imagine feeling any other way?

How would you have chosen? When faced with these kinds of difficult decisions, many of us get overwhelmed by the possibilities. At which point, we begin to doubt ourselves. And if this self doubt goes on for long enough, we may feel urges to just accept whatever our wise man advises.

What's wrong with doing this? A whole lot, actually. Including that habitually deferring to the opinions of others will eventually turn even the smartest person into a dumb person. I, for one, have seen some very smart folks act really dumb under pressure. Myself included.

Why do we do this? Some of us still feel intimidated by our parents' opinions. This feeling then generalizes to all authority figures. I felt this way for much of my life. Some of us never complete our formal education, so we get intimidated by people who have formal titles and professional degrees. My father, a very smart man, told me he felt like this a lot. Some of us can't bear to admit we do not have an answer, as when we have no answer, we feel stupid. So rather than feel stupid, we act stupid, by offering someone else's answer. Still others can't believe that becoming smart takes time. So they mistake quick answers for being smart.

Smart people may, at times, even experience urges to do these things. They just won't give in to the pressure. Nor will they give up when they feel uncomfortable or get intimidated. Rather, they'll keep on searching no matter how uncomfortable it gets.

Smart people also know *where* to seek truth. They seek it inside themselves. To them, seeking their truth in others feels like letting someone else dress you. Yes, these clothes may fit you fine. But they'll never feel the same as those you choose on your own.

The point is, no one can tell you what your personal truth should be. Nor should you be asking anyone to give this to you. At best, all you'll learn is their personal truth. At worst, you'll feel even more dumb and lost.

Fortunately the friends I mentioned have learned not to do this. In fact, at one point, I saw John risk insulting a doctor by schmoozing in the hallway with this doctor's nurses. He wanted to get the real scoop on cochlear implants and which doctor to go with. And he did. And as I watched him do this, I welled up with tears. Imagine living your life this way—not giving up until you find your personal truth? My friend John does. You can too.

Can Theories Describe the Whole Truth?

One thing to keep in mind as you read this or any book is that a lot of things sound good in theory, but don't translate well to the real world. Have you ever considered how often this impacts your ability to make decisions, especially those you make in and around health and family? Take for example the decision to follow a doctor's directions regarding a medication. In theory, you should follow your doctor's orders. But in the real world, you need to include yourself in these decisions.

For instance, consider the decision to take cholesterol medication. For decades doctors have been advising folks to take a statin. Why? Because lowering cholesterol is supposed to lower your chances for heart disease and stroke. And statins do a good job lowering cholesterol. According to some pretty smart people however, statistics collected over the past couple of decades don't always translate into the kinds of improvements in the rates of heart disease and stroke most folks hope for. And some folks even feel worse.

So should you take a statin? Don't ask me. I'm no M.D. And by all means, don't take what I've just said to be me claiming to know the whole truth about statins. I will admit however that I chose to not take a statin, this despite my cholesterol being somewhat high. What made me decide to do this? I did my homework. I went to my doctor several times including for blood tests (I collected facts). Then per his advice, I tried a number of natural remedies (I got personal experience). I also read up on people's theories about cholesterol (I explored ideas). And I also exercised and meditated a lot more (I focused on my spiritual self).

The good news? After three months, my overall cholesterol dropped 35 points. The bad news? Four months later, my number had climbed back up almost to where I'd started, this despite my continued efforts. As it turns out, I'm genetically prone to high cholesterol. If I do something to lower it, my body just makes more.

Why tell you this? In theory, this treatment should have worked. But in the real world, it seems, I'm a strange duck. Oh, isn't that the truth. And while I in no way recommend you ignore your doctor's advice, I do urge you to do more than just take his or her word as the whole truth. Go out and investigate, and find your own personal truth.

Can Facts Be the Whole Truth?

Another thing to keep in mind as you read this series of books is how facts affect you. Some folks see facts as the main element of truth. Others blow them off entirely. Take the side effects listed on medication labels. Some folks read these side effects and refuse to take a medication. To them, it's not worth the risk. Others choose to disregard these warnings and treat their doctor's reassurances as if they come straight from God.

Curiously, drug company disclosures, or the lack thereof, play a big part in both these decisions. Admittedly, these disclosures can sound pretty frightening. In the real world, though, do most or even many people experience these side effects? Well, this depends. The minor ones, yes. But the more serious ones? Of course not.

The truth here? It's hard to know. Which is why some folks see drug company disclosures as a literal truth and choose not to take a medication, while others choose to ignore these warnings and base their decision on their relationship with their doctor.

In the first case, folks mistake a factual truth for a whole truth. In the second, folks avoid the facts entirely. Will either of these paths lead to a personal truth? Definitely not. Despite this, many people make decisions this way all the time.

Do Whole Truths Even Exist?

Yet another thing to keep in mind as you read this book is that many of us assume every question has an answer. An ultimate answer. *The* answer. Moreover we believe these answers can and should be measurable and lasting. No less than Einstein himself was of this opinion and in fact spent much of his life trying to prove it. Hence his famous remark discounting uncertain answers—"I can't believe God plays dice."

Who are we to think we know more than Einstein? Who are we not to if we disagree with him? Moreover when it comes to personal truth, it turns out, no human being has more potential than another. Some of us just get born with more access to this potential, which then gives us more access to certain kinds of truth.

Are there ultimate answers to questions? As it turns out, no. Not even in physics is this true. We'll talk more about why in Book III. Why mention this? Because many of us believe such answers exist. So we drive ourselves crazy looking for them. Then when we don't find them, we become discouraged and feel lost. Worse yet, sometimes, we end up feeling so bad that we stop believing in ourselves.

What people overlook here is that personal truths change. Thus what we should be looking for is what is true for us *at this particular time.* The point is, because personal truths change, there can never be one right answer. Only a right answer for now. Sadly most of us never learn to accept this.

We then end up believing in some pretty strange ideas. For example, take the idea that we each have a soul mate. Or at least, someone whom is "right" for us, our ultimate other-half. People who believe this idea frequently end up unhappy, insisting they have settled. Yet rationally, this idea is crazy. No relationship is perfect. Factually, it's obviously untrue as well. All people struggle and fight. Empirically, life doesn't support this belief either. Real happily-ever-aftering stories occur rarely, if at all.

And spiritually? Despite evidence to the contrary, some people never stop looking.

How about you? Do you believe in soul mates? If so, then ask yourself this. Have you personally ever met a couple to whom happily-ever-aftering has happened *in a lasting way*? Me? In my twenty plus years as a therapist, I've not observed a single case. Nor do I expect to. Why do some of us continue to believe in such an absurd idea then? Because like Einstein, we refuse to believe that psychological hard work and spiritual persistence will not lead us to an ultimate answer. In his case, to a unified field theory. In our case, to our perfect mate.

Ironically, there is a perfect person for you—the one who is reading this book. You. But only if you can honor yourself and your personal truth. Moreover, while Socrates was right when he said that the unexamined life is not worth living, at the same time, nothing kills people's chances for a good life more than constantly searching for something which doesn't exist—an ultimate truth. So yes, I agree with Socrates—the unexamined life is not worth living. But the over examined life is just as worthless. My point? Personal truths are not ultimate truths. We are, after all, only human.

What Makes Something a Personal Truth?

Now we're going to discuss personal truth in the everyday sense of truth. What is it? Simply put, personal truth is *anything which affects us personally*. Big things. Small things. Any and all things. If it affects us as people, it involves personal truth.

How often do we seek personal truth? Each time we ask or answer a personal question. What do I want for dinner? What time do I want to get up? Which movie do I want to see tonight? Who do I think will win the series?

Why don't we call these questions, seeking personal truth?

Because most of us see truth as a big thing, and these questions are trivial. Then again, if someone were to ask you one of these questions then ignore your answer, you would probably get quite annoyed. You might even make a big deal out of their doing this, perhaps by complaining, "why ask if you didn't want to hear my answer?" To which they might respond, "why are you making such a big deal out of nothing?"

Is it no big deal when someone ignores us though? Of course not. And while these kinds of questions are indeed ordinary, our reactions reveal their true value. Small questions do indeed matter, much more than we normally admit. Thus any and all questions which affect us personally should be seen as seeking personal truth.

With Personal Truth, Things Can Add Up Differently

A second thing to know about personal truth is that where and when you seek it changes your answer. This includes not only questions about personal choices like what to wear and which movie to see. It also includes questions which have seemingly obvious answers, like the answer to two plus two. And yes, in theory, two plus two does have one right answer—four. But personally?

To see what I mean, let's say these two plus two "things" were four things which you could not always add together, two close friends plus two casual friends, for example. What would your personal truth be here? Would you have two friends plus two friends equaling four friends, or would you have two close friends and two casual friends which is two *and* two, not two *plus* two?

Am I being picayune? Perhaps. Even so, my point still stands. Finding your personal truth requires more than theoretical rationale and logic (your ideas). It also requires clear facts, honest feelings, and personal stories as well. For instance, if you needed people to vote for you, four friends might sound pretty good. But if you were in trouble and needed someone to call, you'd likely see these four friends as only two.

When it comes to personal truth then, strange as it sounds, seemingly trivial differences can make a big difference. Do you have two close friends and two casual friends? Or do you have four friends? Having a good life requires you pay attention to these kinds of details, as personal truth doesn't always add up the same.

With Personal Truth, You Can't Leave Things Out

Speaking of how things can add up differently, this might be a good time to remind you that it takes four wise men to make a personal truth—a *rationalist* wise man, a *materialist* wise man, an *empirical* wise man, and a *spiritual* wise man. As well as the four great truths these four wise men provoke in you—ideas, facts, stories, and feelings.

Why do we need all four wise men's truths?

Imagine doing your taxes and that you're entitled to a refund. But you leave some deductions out. You had the receipts, but you overlooked them. Crap! Or that you're baking chocolate chip cookies and they usually turn out great but you forget to put in salt. It was right there on the counter, but you forgot. Whoa! Or you're writing a paper on dodo birds (raphus cucullatus) and you've researched this paper to the max but you forgot to mention they're extinct. Oh, boy! Or it's your first wedding anniversary and you knew it but forgot to get flowers. So you wish her happy anniversary and try to wing it. Screwed!

This is what happens to us when we overlook a wise man. Crap! I left out some important *facts*. Whoa! I skipped a step in the *story*. Oh, boy! I missed the main *idea*. Screwed! I forgot my wife's *feelings*. And since, by nature, we are programmed to leave at least one wise man out, these things tend to happen a lot. So yes, your wife won't necessarily divorce you. Nor will your professor always give you a failing grade. But you may feel squirrelly and defensive. And you won't find much personal truth.

The point is, truths become personal truths only when we include all the parts. Leave something out and you'll know it. Include all the parts and you'll know that too. This, in fact, is the best way to recognize a personal truth. If it feels personally satisfying and complete, then it's a personal truth. If not, then you've probably left something out.

Summarizing What I've Said About Personal Truth

At this point, I realize I've told you a lot. So let me recap.

Personal truths are whole truths and whole truths satisfy. So why don't we seek whole truths more? Mainly because of how the word *truth* affects us when we hear it. In reality, each time we ask a question, we seek personal truth. But because the word *truth* sounds so grand, and because we habitually defer to the truths of others, rarely if ever do we call what we're seeking *truth*.

What difference does this make?

In the short run, probably not much. Over time, though, it can make a big difference. For instance, consider how we respond when people fuss about what we consider dumb questions. Often, we judge them pretty harshly. This includes not only questions about things we feel they should know because they're important. It also includes small everyday decisions like when to eat and what to wear.

For example, take the stereotypical wife's complaint—*he never listens to me*. Now ask yourself what she's complaining about. Is she complaining about what her husband thinks of God and country? Or is she complaining about how he never hears her requests to take out the garbage?

What about the typical fourteen year old's complaint—that her parents never listen to her. As a therapist, I've heard kids complain about this more times than I can count. So are they complaining because their parents don't care about their health and grades? Or are they complaining because their parents don't listen to them when they say they *need* to go to the mall or *can't* wear last year's jeans or *don't* want their little sister tagging along?

Can you see where this is going? By calling your personal questions "seeking personal truth," you become more self aware. You also get better at responding to other people's personal questions, and this can improve your relationships. In addition, you get to feel less ashamed when you don't have answers. Truth is a big deal and we don't always know the truth. And you also improve your self worth by treating the small details in your life as important.

What about when we ask the more serious questions though? Don't we usually pay more attention to them? Questions like which school would give your child the best chance to succeed? Is it a good time to ask for a raise? How can you know if your fiancé will make a good mother? Which diet will help you to lose weight?

What should you be looking for in a career anyway—security, challenge, financial reward, personal freedom? And what can you do to avoid getting cancer—eat right, exercise more, take supplements? Certainly these kinds of questions are more serious, and personal. And in general, we do pay more attention to them. Even so, most people see them more as conjecture about what they *should* be doing than as efforts to find personal truth.

What about the questions we raise during major life changes? Do we realize we're seeking personal truth then? When a death occurs? When we consider getting married? When we lose a job? When a child is born? Surprisingly, many people fail to see even these kinds of questions as seeking personal truth. For them, truth is something only science or religion can tell us. Why am I alive? Do I have a purpose? Is there life after death? Is there a meaning to my suffering? Even with intensely personal questions such as these, some folks still don't see themselves seeking personal truth.

The point, of course, is that every question we ask seeks personal truth. Yet even under intensely personal circumstances, most people fail to recognize the importance of seeking their own answers. That this can happen even when faced with decisions like picking a cancer treatment or getting divorced is downright sad. Even here, though, most folks will focus more on finding scientifically or spiritually "right" answers than on finding what feels personally true to them. And they'll more likely seek answers online, from other people, in bookstore self-help aisles, or from television psychologists than from inside themselves.

The good news is, you can change this. You can learn to seek truth in yourself. To do this, you'll need to get better at noticing the significance of your everyday questions. Indeed, the more attention you pay to these questions, and to all people's personal questions really, the more authentic you'll become—at being a friend, a sibling, a parent, a co-worker, and a better human being in general. Moreover, you get all this, not from having answers but rather, from recognizing that all of your questions seek personal truth.

The thing to remember then is that each time you answer a question, you set the bar for your life and relationships. Answer authentically and you raise the bar. Answer mindlessly and you lower it. And of course, if occasionally you fail to do this, it will not make or break most relationships. But fail to do it enough and it just might.

To Find Your Truth, You'll Need a Method

Now we come to one of the main points of this book—the idea that to find your personal truth, you need a method. Why do you need a method? Because without one, finding personal truth is more like trying to win a lottery than living your life consciously. You also need this method for the times wherein you do manage to find the courage to seek your truth only to hear shaming remarks like: "Why do you have to be so difficult?"—"What are you, a trouble maker?"—"Can't you just be like other people?"—"Why reinvent the wheel?"

To be honest, I've always found this strange. We generally admire inventors and explorers. Yet we shame all but the youngest children for wanting to be like them. Historically, even the great philosophers have been shamed for seeking truth. Perhaps this explains why so many of them focused on "defining truth," as in, how to know it when you see it, rather than on how to find it.

René Descartes (my editor tells me it's pronounced, *deh-cart*, not *des-cartes*) was an exception. In 1637, he published his *Discourse on the Method for Directing One's Reason Well and Searching for Truth in the Sciences*, a book in which he describes his method for finding truth. Notable is the idea that Descartes does not include in his book a way to know something is false. Rather he says his method will allow you to either [1] discern the truth about a thing or [2] know you cannot know this truth. This idea—that we cannot know the truth about some things—is among Descartes' most profound. The four wise men's method incorporates this principle as well.

What made Descartes' book significant? For one thing, he tells us he chose to publish his book in French, not Latin, so that women could learn his method. In 1637. Imagine? For another, he tells us we must disregard what we've been taught and trust only what we ourselves discover. Our personal truth. He also tells us we'll need to meditate in order to understand his method. And by *meditate*, he means we'll need to take the time to search our mind for clear and distinct observations based on what we see about what he is saying. He even goes so far as to say some folks may not be able to do this and he is right. However, based on his choice to write in French, what he's actually saying is, if you take your time you'll do fine.

How does Descartes say he arrived at his truths? He tells us it took four steps. Here, I voice them as if he is telling them to you.

❧

1. You must begin with what is clear and distinct, never accepting anything as true without it being so clear and distinct as to exclude all possibility of doubt.

2. You must divide each of the things being examined into as many parts as possible and into as many parts as may be necessary for an adequate solution.

3. You must begin with the parts which are simplest and easiest to know and only then ascend in complexity, assigning an order to all the parts.

4. Finally you must make enumerations so complete and reviews so general that you will be assured you have omitted nothing.

❧

How does Descartes' method compare to the one you'll find in this book?

Students of philosophy get taught that Descartes was a *rationalist*. Descartes in fact supports this impression telling us he trusts only reason. Indeed, he goes to great lengths to discount the reliability of truths derived from other methods, including from empirical observations, from material observations, and from spiritual observations. Yet if you read Descartes' *Rules For The Direction of the Mind*, an unfinished book which predates *Discourse on the Method* by some nine years, you find that what Descartes refers to as rational steps are roughly analogous to the methods I will shortly enumerate here. Descartes simply reframes his steps in words which make them sound like four well-ordered, rational steps.

Please notice I just said *roughly*. Moreover, in no way does the value of the present book depend on finding a literal parallel to Descartes' book. Rather, I mention Descartes' work as it has greatly affected me. As well as to point out that his book contains many curious parallels to what I'm presenting here.

How does the method I'm presenting here parallel Descartes'?

1. Descartes' step 1—that you must feel clear about your direction and focus, roughly parallels the spiritual wise man's method—*a truth must feel emotionally true—you must let go of all you know and trust your intuition to guide you to a starting point.*

2. His step two—that you must divide what you're doing into discernible pieces roughly parallels the method of the materialist wise man—*a truth must be factually true—measurements must be taken.*

3. Descartes' step three—that you must arrange these pieces in a logical order and only then ascend in complexity roughly parallels the method of the empirical wise man—*a truth must be empirically true—these facts must tell a story.*

4. Descartes' step four—that you must derive your conclusions by comprehensively reviewing the entire process roughly parallels the method of the rationalist wise man—*a truth must be rationally true—the pieces of this story must fit together logically.*

Finally, for those interested in exploring these parallels further including Descartes' complete case for why we need a method, I suggest you read Descartes' *Rules For The Direction of the Mind.* Even unfinished, this book remains amazingly clear and relevant. It also serves to clarify his later works, especially the *Discourse on Method,* as well as supporting much of what underlies the present book.

In addition to noting Descartes' book as an historical antecedent to the present work, I would also like to acknowledge how his life has personally inspired me. Like most of us, Descartes felt afraid to speak his personal truth openly. He in fact feared he'd be killed for what he wrote. Despite this fear, eventually, he published his thoughts on how to find truth anyway, in effect, finally disregarding his personal motto, "I advance masked."

I believe we all, at times, feel like Descartes felt—afraid we'll be punished for speaking out. I myself have repeatedly felt this way throughout my life. Thus I admire Descartes for facing his fear and for speaking out. Hopefully this book will inspire you to do the same.

And if someone tries to punish you for speaking out? To me, finding personal truth is our *raison d'être*—our reason for being. Thus I encourage you to do all you can to learn to ask more questions. And if a teacher, or friend, or lover balks at your doing this? Then give them the boot. You deserve people who want to hear, and share, your personal truth.

As for why we need a method, it's simple. Given we're so likely to be shamed, blamed, or punished for speaking out, it's important to be able to report, in a clear and distinct manner, how we arrived at our truth. We may have missed a step. Or we may realize the other person missed hearing one of our steps. Either way, being clear about how you arrive at your truth is part of what makes a truth personal. They're your steps. It's your path. Thus knowing these things is important.

How an Aha Moment Led to This Method

In the next chapter, we'll begin to look at how the four wise men can help you to find your personal truth. Before we do, I need to talk a bit about how I came to know they exist. You see, like Descartes, I spent years trying to find my own truth. Unlike him, though, I was unaware I had been using a method. All this changed one day when I took on a new student and asked myself how I might best teach him. And while the particulars of what I was trying to teach him that day are not relevant, the story of how I came to be teaching him is.

What do I teach? Fourteen or so years ago, I had what many people would call a "spiritual experience." As a result, I began to study, and teach, the nature of such experiences. I soon realized these events hold the key to a lot more than just how we make spiritual discoveries. Not that this is any small thing. But they also hold the key to understanding human nature in general, from how we heal and fall in love, to how we learn and grow.

I also discovered that spiritual experiences have a sort of evil twin, the times wherein we get startled. Moreover, while it's obvious to all that being startled empties the mind, there's something far more insidious that we haven't known about startles—that experiencing this sudden emptiness permanently impairs our ability to mentally visualize things. This is not to say being startled permanently blinds us to everything in life. Only to a select few things. But because we record not only these few things but also the fractal patterns which led to our going blind, these blind spots quickly spread through our mind like psychological viruses, impairing our ability to learn, change, grow, love, and heal in these areas of life.

Can you see the implications of what I've just said? Being startled wounds our ability to mentally visualize things. Thus our personal problems come not so much from our symptoms (depression, ADHD, anxiety) or painful acts (rage, lashing out, overeating), nor even from painful events (being raped, robbed, being in a car accident). Rather, they come from *the impaired visual abilities which lead us to be unable to avoid these things.*

This explains why we need to be able to see the entire map of the mind. Whenever we can't manage to see the whole map, we know we have encountered a blind spot. Thus because being startled damages our ability to see this map, knowing what a whole map looks like holds the key to a healthy life.

Can you see what makes this discovery about startles so important? For the first time, we can empirically define, test for, and understand the nature of our wounds. Unfortunately, because blankness, like all holes, in and of itself cannot be seen, you may have a hard time believing these blind spots exist. Or that we can't just override them with logic. Know we'll talk at length about this hypothesis throughout this series of books.

We'll also talk about how this discovery allows us to empirically define healing. So what is it? *Healing* is *the act of restoring our lost visual abilities.* Not coincidently healing events are no different in nature from those we have been calling epiphanies. In other words, if being startled into blankness is the essence of a wounding event, then what happens in healing events should be the converse of this. And it is. Amazement— awe and wonder—becoming hyper-visual. Sounds like how we describe epiphanies, doesn't it?

This same discovery also allows us to define learning as well. *Learning* is *the act of creating new visual abilities.* Here we see yet another class of events we should be calling epiphanies. Moreover, because we feel awed, inspired, and amazed whenever we learn to visualize things, and because these feelings are what lead to our falling in love, we can now define the nature of love itself. *Love* is *the experience of becoming able to visualize the beauty in life.* Yet another class of epiphanies.

I find this last idea particularly salient. We fall in love each time we learn to see beauty. This means love includes not only the things we label "true love," like the love of a spouse or your day old daughter's smile. It also includes the love of things like your new yellow sports car or the diamond ring you've been dreaming of. All these experiences are indeed true love. Thus our problems with love stem more from our inability to define what it is than with managing to get it. And we can find our wounds just by exploring the things we can't manage to love.

How Another Aha Led to the Four Wise Men's Map

As for how I discovered the map, fast forward some twelve years. It was a Sunday morning and my new student showed up promptly at 11. Since I and my other students have spent more than a decade exploring how aha moments and startles affect human nature, and since my new student had joined our group only recently, I offered to tutor him inbetween groups.

In addition, this fellow had previously shared with me that he suffers from a learning disability. From this, I knew he and I might struggle a bit during our tutoring session. Moreover as I have personally committed to never suffer without gain, I saw in our potential struggle a great possibility to learn more about how people learn.

As we started, then, I remember telling him I was not exactly sure how best to begin. We then sat across from each other on my living room floor and I remember writing the word *fractal* on a 3 x 5 card. I then placed this card on the floor and asked him what came to mind. We then proceeded to discuss everything we knew about fractals, card by card.

Since everything I do is based on fractals, for me, this encompassed quite a lot. Including a difficult concept called emergence, which is what chaos theorists and complexity scientists call unexpected events and I call spiritual experiences. Being these events are filled with uncertainty, this stuff can be tough to understand. Unless you know the key to living with uncertainty, in which case, it becomes slightly less tough.

What seemed to help that day was that I limited what I wrote to one idea per card. I then intuitively arranged these cards in what later turned out to be a series of interrelated continuums. In no time at all, we had dozens of cards on the floor. And to our surprise, both of us could recall not only what was said, but also how it was said—the actual process.

Then, in the midst of admiring our work, I had an aha. I realized that what had inadvertently been unfolding on my floor was the method by which I had been making my discoveries. I also realized this method had many similarities to Descartes' method for finding truth. Thus these cards were not so much documenting the ideas I was teaching my student as they were revealing the inner workings of my mind.

Five hours later, we stopped, both of us thoroughly overwhelmed. My floor was covered in 3 x 5 cards—our brains were totally full. Then that evening, my student e-mailed me with yet another surprise. He said he'd never retained so much, this despite the fact that we'd not slowed down once in the whole five hours. Ideas, stories, facts, and feelings had just poured out of us both.

Days later, I made the drawing which appears on the second page of this chapter. In essence, it's just a fancy copy of what had appeared on my living room floor that day. Then a week later, I introduced this map to my group, along with the idea that all knowledge derives from a synthesis of the wisdom of four wise men—the rationalist, the materialist, the empiricist, and the spiritualist.

Within days, I'd also begun to develop the game which you'll learn about later, a simple tool you can use to determine which wise men you trust and which you tend to ignore. And while this game is but the prelude to finding your personal truth, still, because the idea of the four wise men manages to so completely describe the principles and concepts underlying all of human nature, playing this simple game can put you closer to every truth you seek.

Perhaps what surprises me most though is something one of my therapy practice clients said to me a few days after that meeting with my student. When I showed my client my first drawing of the map, he asked if I realized what I had discovered. I told him, I thought I had. A moment later, though, he surprised me by telling me he thought I should be careful—that like Einstein living to regret having discovered $e=mc^2$ because it led to the atom bomb, that I might live to feel similar feelings. Why? He said because what was contained in that drawing was not just a map of *my* mind. It was the fractal for artificial intelligence—a map of *all* human minds. And that it could be misused and potentially do harm.

Can he be right? To be honest, I don't know. For one thing, it's too early to tell—I've not gathered enough information. For another, I am not a scientist by profession. Nor do I wish to be. But when I see the degree to which playing the game even once can change a person's life, it makes me wonder. Thus I have to admit, this warning has given me reason to pause.

At the same time, I believe there is an inherent goodness in all human beings, a wonderful natural light which grows dim when we stop seeking personal truth. Thus even if there is reason for concern, the very reason for worry may be the antidote itself. I also believe that the same free will that can lead to hatred can lead to love. Thus while the possibility exists that some folks may indeed choose to misuse what I'm offering, I choose to believe goodness will win out.

Whatever the truth about the underlying nature of what I've discovered, I want you to know my intentions for writing this book are clear. You have it in you to become a genius. You have only to be taught how. Moreover I believe the best use for this genius would be to create new ways for people to love each other. Including yourself. Thus I hope and pray you'll use what you learn here to better our world.

Ultimately then, this series of books; *Finding Personal Truth (in the too-much-information age)*, offers a useful, doable, and teachable method for finding your truth. What kind of truth? Any truth. This is possible because what underlies this method is a fractal map of the mind. And a method so easily learned that just about anyone can use it.

Notes Written in the Margins of Chapter One

On Reinventing the Wheel

Books such as this one often include things like sidebars and footnotes. I, myself, most times, find these side trips distracting at best and downright confusing at worst. At the same time, I do like reading more about the parts of a book I find interesting or confusing. Thus at the end of each chapter, you'll find I've included what amount to footnotes, sidebars, notes I myself would have chosen to write in the margins, and references to further reading.

In part, I've chosen to do this as it mirrors what I do with books in my personal life. Thus despite my mother's frequent admonishments to never deface a book by writing in it, I have come to love writing in the margins of books. I see this as my way to dialogue with the author of said book. More important, in the process, I get to treat myself as being equal to the author of said book, at least with regard to my ability to discern truth.

Am I always equal? As a human being, yes. I say this knowing others frequently know far more than I by virtue of their educations. At the same time, I believe no one learns truth from parroting another's truth no matter how great the teacher. Thus despite the obvious virtues inherent in advising us to not reinvent the wheel, I believe this counsel misses the mark. By all means, feel free to retrace the steps of any teacher from which you may wish to learn. But do this step by step and include yourself in the process, only then comparing the teacher's conclusions to your own.

What I'm saying is, human beings become wheel makers only by reinventing wheels. Failing this, at best, we become mere parrots of other people's truth. Moreover, while I personally encourage you to seek whatever truth your heart desires, at the same time, I recommend you never take a teacher's summary as the proof for a truth.

Worse yet is attempting to find the truth in a teacher's words second hand. By this I mean, reading those dreadful analyses wherein a so-called expert bores us to tears by endlessly dissembling a teacher's thoughts into mind-sized bites. In the end, this can only lead to misunderstandings and confusion, a lesson I learned the hard way only after years of trying to ingest these so called shortcuts to the truth.

For instance, I, for years, thought Freud a cold and arrogant prick. Then one day I realized I should at least try to read the prick in his own words. At which point, I naively drove to a bookstore thinking I'd just buy one of his books, never realizing my entire understanding would rest on the skill of the translator I chose. Freud wrote in German. I do not read German. Duh. Imagine my surprise then when I compared translations to see which would be most readable only to discover, to my dismay, that these translations often differed so greatly as to make Freud's intent unknowable. They literally make Freud's words appear to have been authored by different people. Which in truth, they were. It had just never occurred to me the degree to which these "auxiliary" authors can unintentionally obfuscate a source.

In the end, I fell in love with yet another man who risked all to put in writing his personal truth. More so when I later read a letter Freud wrote to a man who had originally been one of his greatest detractors, Fredrik Willem van Eeden, the originator of Lucid Dreaming. In this letter, Freud admits to van Eeden that he had based his book, *Interpretation of Dreams*, on his own life experiences. After which it seems van Eeden warmed to Freud, perhaps much like we warm to similarly brave souls.

My point is, please don't take anyone's word for what is true. Doing this means you'll miss the chance to discover your own personal truth. This includes the truths of both translators of famous teachers and aspiring wise men like me. Thus I encourage you to take the time to reinvent what I'm saying in your own words. Only then can you hope to discover what is true for you. Including that it might just turn out that I am not a cold arrogant prick either. One can only hope.

On My Choice to Use the Phrase Wise *Men*

Throughout the book, I refer to the source of truth as the Four Wise Men. To some, my choice to use the word *men* may make me appear sexist. Please know I in no way intend to give the reader this impression. Moreover I fully acknowledge women are just as good at finding wisdom as men. Sometimes, they're even better.

I also delight in knowing that if you look up the word *philosophy*, you'll find it comes from two Greek sources, one of them being the word, *sophia*, the early Greek's way to refer to the source of wisdom. Sophia was the goddess of wisdom. Hence the *sophy* part of the word philosophy is named after a woman, not a man. At the same time, I am so tired of hearing rants wherein men and women are admonished for not using politically correct language. Whitewash the world and you cover up the truth. Moreover when people stilt their ideas with artificially created equality, it destroys something beautiful. Furthermore, this is so unnecessary as it's entirely possible to respect people's gender, race, religion, ethnicity and so on while at the same time honoring people's differences.

As for my choice to use the phrase *wise men*, I see "compensatory sexism" as being as destructive to truth seeking as sexism itself. What should I call them, wise *persons*? Moreover, as my dad taught me, two wrongs do not make a right. Thus in the end, I've chosen to use this phrase more for the images it conjures up in the minds of both men and women than as my taking a stand that men are smarter than women and or know more truth. They don't. I'm simply piggybacking onto an already venerated tradition.

Still feel mad at me for using the word *men*? Then so be it. I can honor your anger. In the mean time, please do try to honor me for wanting to voice my book from the eyes and heart of my personal truth. This truth includes the idea that while diversity never fails to interest me, at the same time, whitewashing, like mistaking parroting for true learning, never fails to make me want to puke. And it's hard to seek truth when you're feeling sick.

A Few Thoughts About the Idea that Stress Causes Illness

In the next chapter, we'll talk a lot about the importance of words, specifically, about how the words we use determine the meanings we assign to our ideas. Moreover, while it is surely premature to discuss the idea that stress causes illness, because I've introduced you to the idea that our wounds are mental blind spots, it might be a good idea to briefly discuss one of the main properties of these blind spots—*stress*.

What is stress? To see, consider what it would be like to go through life blind. Even doing ordinary acts, like walking across a room, could cause you to feel stress. Now consider what it is like to temporarily go blind, for instance, during an argument when you lose control. Has this ever happened to you? If so, then you know you can't picture anything in these moments. Nor can you picture anything afterwards when you try to access these moments. You literally go blank inside.

The point is, it's these mental blind spots that cause us to bang into things, and the fear that we'll do this is what causes most of our stress. We're bracing for the bang. Moreover, it's not hard to see how repeatedly trying to do something while blind would affect your health over time.

In general, then, stress is what we feel whenever we do something blind. We fear we may bang into something, so we tense up and brace ourselves, both psychologically and physically. Resentment then generalizes this tenseness into whole categories of stress, and over time, these categories of stress are what lead to illness. More on this later.

A Few Words About the Word *Fractal*

Finally, for those scientifically minded folks who get set off when a person like me uses a word like "fractal," please note that I define this word a bit differently. Moreover, true to the spirit of this book, I've spent more than a decade searching for a personally satisfying way to define this word. The result? Unlike the technically-minded complexity scientists who define this word more by what it does than by what it is (for instance, as a rough or fragmented geometric shape that can be split into parts, each of which is approximately a smaller copy of the whole), I use the manner favored by the ancient Greeks to define this word. I define it by its sine qua non—by it essence. Thus a *fractal* is a "recognizable pattern which always repeats differently."

Why go through so much trouble to define the word *fractal*?

Traditional sciences see linear patterns as the only acceptable proof of truth. In other words, what proves something true to them is that the results repeat the same way every time. In effect, traditional sciences make outcomes such as impeccable logic or statistically meaningful repetitions their holy grail. Thus we can define the kind of truths they seek—linear truths—as "recognizable patterns which always repeat *identically*."

Can you see the difference here? Recognizable patterns which always repeat *differently* (fractal truths) versus recognizable patterns which always repeat *identically* (linear truths). Fractal truths repeat differently. Linear truths repeat identically. Now recall that traditional sciences see linearity as the only acceptable truth. Unfortunately, while meaningful statistics and scientific logic obviously have their place, nothing in the real world is linear. Thus without fractal truths to counterbalance linear truths, our truths remain trapped inside the laboratory.

By juxtaposing linearity with fractility, however, we override this shortcoming. Fractility becomes the proof of truth in the real world, and linearity the proof of truth in theory. We also get a meaningful starting point from which to understand much of what we'll be looking at in this series of books, including a way to see how theoretical and real world truths relate. In addition, we get a legitimately scientific way to define the nature of things, both linear and non linear alike. And we also get to understand the essence of what stumped as great a mind as Einstein—how uncertainty relates to certainty.

So. Are you ready to know more than Einstein knew about truth? Big breath now. Personal truth, here we come.

Resources for Chapter One—Truth Seeking... We All Do It

On Descartes (1596-1650)

Do you have a friend who reads French? Then by all means, consider asking this friend to translate in front of you the parts of Descartes' writings which most interest you. For instance, I asked my friend and editor, Avital, to translate the title of the Discourse on Method from French to English. We then came up with what we see as a more accurate translation for this title than those previously posited. We also spent much time discussing certain words Descartes used, for instance the word *esprit*, without which Descartes' intentions regarding the spiritual side of truth cannot be known.

In lieu of doing this, or as an additional resource, I recommend the following.

Descartes, René. (1985). *The Philosophical Writing of Descartes, Volume 1: Rules for the Direction of the Mind, Discourse on the Method, etc.* (John Cottingham, Robert Stoothoff, Dugald Murdoch, Trans.). New York: Cambridge University Press. (Originally published 1627, 1637) (This is my current favorite for a published translation.)

Descartes, René. (1985). *The Philosophical Writing of Descartes, Volume 2: Meditations on First Philosophy, etc.* (John Cottingham, Robert Stoothoff, Dugald Murdoch, Trans.). New York: Cambridge University Press. (Originally published 1641)

Descartes, René. (1985). *The Philosophical Writing of Descartes, Volume 3: the Correspondence.* (John Cottingham, Robert Stoothoff, Dugald Murdoch, Anthony Kenny, Trans.). New York: Cambridge University Press.

Descartes, René. (2004). *Discourse on Method* and *Meditations on the First Philosophy.* (Veitch, John. Trans.). New York: Barnes and Noble. (This is a good translation against which to compare that of Cottingham, et al.)

Descartes, René. (2001). *Discourse on Method, Optics, Geometry, and Meteorology* (Paul J. Olscamp, Trans.). Indianapolis, IN: Hackett Publishing (Yet another good translation against which to compare that of Cottingham, et al. Worth reading just for the translator's preface.)

Aczel, Amir D. (2005). *Descartes' Secret Notebook.* New York: Broadway Books / Random House. (An interesting sidebar to Descartes, the man, and a good way to sense how he was seen in his time.)

Phemister, Pauline. (2006) *The Rationalists-Descartes, Spinoza and Leibniz.* Cambridge, UK: Polity Press (The type of collegiate analysis I warned you about in the section on reinventing the wheel. Perhaps this is why it costs so much?)

On Cholesterol

As is often the case with things science tells us are true, in the real world, there is always more to know. Case in point. While I was writing this chapter, results from a recent two year study on the effects of one particular statin were published. This study, which included over 17,000 people, showed that this statin does indeed improve people's rates of heart disease and stroke. Significantly. The thing is, they attribute these improvements to that this drug reduces something in addition to cholesterol—CRP levels. Thus while this news is indeed positive, it also points to that cholesterol may not be the only culprit. CRP levels may be part of the problem. More important, in no way does this study address the potential risks anecdotally reported with regard to statins and losses in mental acuity.

This said, here are a few sources I found interesting.

Taubes, Gary. (2007). *Good Calories, Bad Calories, Challenging the Conventional Wisdom on Diet, Weight Control, and Disease.* New York: Alfred A. Knopf / Random House. (Yet another brave soul who has risked putting his truth in writing. I admire Taubes and love the way he clearly describes the historical antecedents and factual evidence behind our fears of both cholesterol and foods containing fats.)

O'Riordan, Michael. (2008). "The side effects of statins: Heart healthy and head harmful?" *HeartWire / theHeart.org, February 12.* <http://www.theheart.org/article/843115.do>. (Reading this and the three references which follow surprised the heck out of me. Prior to reading these articles, I had posited a connection between the substance which feeds our brains—fat—and cognitive agility. Being as I have high levels of lipids in my blood, if true, then cholesterol could have a good side. For me, the jury is still out. Still, it makes me wonder, especially about those things which we're told have no good side. Does cholesterol have a good side? It must. But since it's in our bodies, it's up to us to discover it.)

Beck, Melinda. (2008). "Can a Drug That Helps Hearts Be Harmful to the Brain?" *Wall Street Journal.* February 12. <http://online.wsj.com/article/SB120277403869360595.html?mod=fpa_editors_picks>.

Fallon, Sally & Mary G. Enig PhD. (2004). "Dangers of Statin Drugs: What You Haven't Been Told About Popular Cholesterol-Lowering Medicines." *Wise Traditions in Food, Farming and the Healing Arts, the quarterly magazine of the Weston A. Price Foundation.* Spring. <http://www.westonaprice.org/moderndiseases/statin.html>.

Mercola, Joseph DO. (2008). "The Truth About Cholesterol-Lowering Drugs (Statins), Cholesterol and Health." *Take Control of your Health, The World's Most Popular Natural Health Newsletter.* <http://www.mercola.com/article/statins.htm>.

Kowalski, Robert E. (2004). *The New 8-Week Cholesterol Cure.* New York: HarperCollins Publishers. (This is my favorite book on managing cholesterol. Having survived—and learned from—two bypass operations, Kowalski is no dummy. Good information for all people, including me. Indeed, during the course of writing this book, it helped me to lower my cholesterol by over seventy points. All this without medications.)

On Freud (1856-1939)

Freud, Sigmund. (2005, 1915). *The Interpretation of Dreams.* (A. W. Brill, Trans.). New York: Barnes & Noble. (Original work published 1899).

Freud, Sigmund. (1999). *The Interpretation of Dreams.* (Joyce Crick, Trans.). Oxford, UK: Oxford University Press. (I love this book. I only wish there were better translations. The first one is adequate, as is the second. Best would be to get a German speaking friend and an early German edition and translate it together. You also might find doing this quite enjoyable.)

Ellenberger, Henri F. (1970). *The Discovery of the Unconscious, The History and Evolution of Dynamic Psychiatry.* New York: Basic Books / Perseus Books. (This is my absolute favorite book on the historical development of talk therapy, as well as on the lives of those involved, including Freud. I warn you though, like my books, it may take you several years to read it. Well worth the effort though. I never tire of going back to it.)

Rooksby, Robert & Sybe, Terwee. (1990). "Freud, van Eeden and Lucid Dreaming." *Lucidity Letter, Vol. 9. 2.* Waverly, Iowa: Waverly Publishing.

van Eeden, Frederik. (1913). "A Study of Dreams." *Proceedings of the Society for Psychical Research,* Vol. 26, <http://www.lucidity.com/vanEeden.html>.

On Einstein (1879-1955)

We'll have much to discuss about this amazing man in coming chapters. We will in fact return to him and his ideas again and again. For those for whom references are an important accompaniment to the present chapter though, I suggest the following. Know it is delightfully written and historically personal. All in all a good read.

Lindley, David. (2007, 2008). *Uncertainty-Einstein, Heisenberg, Bohr, and the Struggle For the Soul of Science.* New York: Doubleday / First Anchor Books.

On Being Startled and Stress

Anyone who makes discoveries makes them based on what has been posited before them, even if what has been posited is ultimately found to be flawed or incomplete. Indeed, much of what I have discovered derives directly from my finding flaws in the midst of what are otherwise astute observations. Likewise, I'm sure those who come after me will benefit from applying this same flaw-finding process to my work.

This said, I wish to mention two books which, by provoking this process in me, led me to have several aha moments during the writing of this chapter.

Pervin, Lawrence A. (2002). *Current Controversies and Issues in Personality.* New York: John Wiley & Sons, Inc. (Pervin, and this book in particular, never fails to provoke new questions in me, my thoughts on how stress and placebos connect, for one. In fact, my copy is so filled with notes written in the margins that I feel as if he and I have been having an ongoing conversation for years now. Indeed, no one interested in human nature should omit this book from their reading list. This is solidly well thought out commentary on the major theorists of our day. A must read.)

Harmon-Jones, Eddie & Jennifer S. Beer. (2009). *Methods in Social Neuroscience.* New York: Guilford Press. (One of the main themes I'll be presenting throughout my books is my hypothesis that being startled is what causes wounds. Several chapters of the Harmon-Jones & Beer book offer neurological support for this hypothesis. Moreover, an idea I'll propose toward the end of Book III is that, to be considered a legitimate scientific hypothesis, you must find corroborating evidence for this hypothesis in at least eight dissimilar areas of study. With regard to my hypothesis that being startled causes wounds, I consider the Harmon-Jones & Beer book one of these eight.)

Chapter 2

Words and Truth—Meet the Four Wise Men

Learning to See the Wise Men's Four Truths

Okay. So as I've told you, there are four wise men—each with a truth—and to find your personal truth, you need all four. But who are these four wise men, and why make such a big deal out of their truths?

In a moment, we'll address these questions, along with what keeps us from seeing these four tricksters. Before we do, I need to bring your attention back to something I mentioned in the previous chapter—the idea that we all get deceived by at least one wise man. The thing is, while being deceived by a wise man does prevent us from finding our truth, the wise men claim they mean us no harm and that they do this only because we are naive. And we are. Especially when we seek our truth from others. My point? Be patient. And persistent. And you will learn to find your truth.

In all seriousness, we're only talking about four truths. How hard can learning to see them be? Well, considering how most dictionaries define the word *facts*, I'm not sure. Of the fourteen I consulted, none define this word as anything other than as something true or something done. What makes something true? They don't say. Nor do they say what makes something done. Thus no dictionary actually defines the word *fact*. Ironic, don't you think?

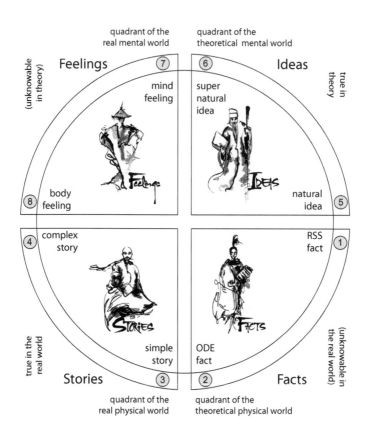

The Four Great Truths
(© 2007 Steven Paglierani   The Center for Emergence)

quadrant of the   quadrant of the
real mental world   theoretical mental world

Feelings   Ideas

(unknowable in theory)   true in theory

mind feeling   super natural idea

body feeling   natural idea

complex story   RSS fact

simple story   ODE fact

true in the real world   (unknowable in the real world)

Stories   Facts

quadrant of the   quadrant of the
real physical world   theoretical physical world

And the word *ideas*? How well do dictionaries define this word? Here again, you'll find, they offer little help. What they do say is that ideas are something mental. An opinion. Or a conviction. Or an estimation. Or a notion. Or a sentiment. Or an impression. Or a plan. Obviously, then, ideas can mean a heck of a lot of things. But what makes something an idea? Again, they do not say.

How about the word *stories*? Do dictionaries do any better here? Admittedly, this time, they do—a story is a narrative event. But stories can also be fabrications, and allegations, and jokes. Which is it? Like facts and ideas, I guess we're just supposed to know.

Worst of all is the way dictionaries define the word *feelings*. Talk about being unclear. Is a feeling, a physical thing? An emotion? An opinion? A hunch? Is it mental? A vague impression? A state of consciousness? An intuited guess? According to most dictionaries, a feeling can be any of these things. So which is it? Again, I guess we're just supposed to know.

Okay. So dictionaries don't define these four words too well. Is this really that important? Don't we all know what these words mean? Well, let me ask you. What makes a fact *scientific*? For that matter, isn't science based on facts? If you think you know, then you might want to read Ludwik Fleck's 1935 monograph, *Genesis and Development of a Scientific Fact*. Do facts get born and then develop? According to Fleck, they do. Likewise Thomas Kuhn who mentions Fleck in the preface of his world changing 1962 book—*The Structure of Scientific Revolutions*.

Still think you know what these four words mean? Then let me ask you. Are *facts* and *ideas* the same? Few people, if any, would say they are. Yet we frequently say things like that so and so is the best man on the team, then follow this with *that's a fact*.

Setting aside for a moment how true this statement may be, whether so and so is indeed the best man on the team is not a fact. It's an opinion. We'll look at why in the section on ideas. Likewise, in the section on feelings, we'll look at another common mix-up, how we often mistake "the idea of feelings" for the feelings themselves.

For instance, when you say you *hate* getting up in the morning, is this hate a feeling or an idea? If, as you say these words, you feel hatred, then it's a feeling. If you don't, then it's an idea.

That we mix-up ideas and feelings, and mistake ideas for facts, does not surprise me. Even a cursory look through a few dictionaries reveals this. That we rarely if ever notice we do this does surprise me though. Especially when we invest so much time trying to figure out what is true.

How the Wise Men Disguise Your Bank Balance

Does it sound like I'm making too big a deal out of how we define these four words? And why call them, the "four great truths?" Well would you believe not having clear definitions for these four words even affects your ability to manage your money? It does. And to demonstrate, we're going to look at a situation some folks find easy, and others near incomprehensible—determining how much you have in your checking account. On the surface, this should be a no-brainer. After all, your bank balance is a fact. Or is it?

In reality, like all personal truths, to figure this out, you need input from all four wise men. You need facts, feelings, stories, and ideas. Does this sound crazy? Well, let's see. What is your balance anyway? Do you know? Most folks don't. And while most people do have an idea of how much money they have, obviously, when it comes to checking accounts, an idea is not enough.

What about you? If you wanted to know how much you have in your checking account, which wise man's truth would you use? Your *factual* bank balance, as in, the ATM number? Your *rational* bank balance, as in, the ATM number plus any unprocessed deposits, minus any outstanding checks. Or would you use your *empirical* bank balance? That is, your rent is due next week. So for the past few weeks, you've subtracted $400 from your check register each week, in order to account for what you'll need. This means your empirical balance is the ATM number, plus any unprocessed deposits, minus any outstanding checks, minus the fake $400 subtractions in your register.

Perhaps, though, you favor your *spiritual* bank balance. Meaning what exactly? Well, God knows what you're feeling about this incredibly convoluted mess of additions and subtractions. Good that you have enough money to pay your rent? Bad that your semi-annual car insurance payment is due in six weeks? Depressed because everything you deposit into your account seems to come out as fast as it goes in? Confident about how well you've managed your money lately?

Are you beginning to see why some folks have a hard time balancing their checkbooks? And if determining your personal truth about your bank balance is this complicated, what does this mean about knowing yourself? At the same time, perhaps I'm making this sound worse than it is. Indeed, Paul Newman may have summed it up pretty well in the 1967 film, *Cool Hand Luke*, when he said: "what we've got here is a failure to communicate." No shit. We have indeed been failing to communicate.

Moreover the problem is not that we've been making too little effort. It's that most of us can't tell a fact from a fart, let alone know what is true.

Am I making truth seeking sound hopeless? Not to worry. After all, we're only talking about four kinds of truth—facts, stories, ideas, and feelings. Moreover, while we all struggle with these words at times, if you can name them, you can learn what they are.

The key, of course, lies in understanding this chapter's theme—knowing how personal truths come into being. You see, all personal truths begin life in the same way—as the materialist wise man's truth—as facts. And as you're about to learn, there are only two kinds of facts. We then arrange these facts in sequences and in doing so, write our stories—the empirical wise man's truth. Here again, there are only two kinds of stories.

Next we generalize what we see in groups of stories, and this is where the rationalist wise man's truth—ideas—come from. Again, there are two kinds of ideas. Finally, when we exceed our capacity to describe what we've experienced with ideas, facts, and stories, we experience the spiritual wise man's truth—the "beyond words" truth—feelings. Two kinds here, too.

Does this sound like a lot to learn? As you'll soon find out, it is. However, if you take your time and read slowly, I'm sure you'll do fine. And if you get bored or lose your way? Then try retracing your steps. Then, when you're comfortable, start working your way forward again.

Above all, keep in mind that no one learns the whole truth. "Whole" truths don't exist, remember? At the same time, if you persevere and seek encouragement and feedback, you can learn to find your truth. Given you can trust yourself.

Okay. Ready to learn how to tell a fact from a fart? Here we go.

P.S. This chapter has turned out to be quite long. Know I agonized over whether to split it into four chapters or keep it all together. I mention this only as I want to be sure you credit yourself for all the work you're about to do. In other words, despite the conservative chapter numbering scheme I've chosen to use, by the time you've finished this chapter, you'll have read what amount to five ordinary chapters, not two. Five long ass chapters, at that.

When you get done then, please give yourself time to let what you've read sink in. And do take a few moments to remind yourself of who you are—a truly brave soul.

Know you can learn all of what's in this book. Just believe in yourself and you will succeed.

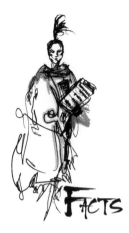

FACTS

Where are facts true? (the horizontal axis position)	*Only* **in theory** (facts are unknowable in the real world)
In what time do facts exist? (temporal frame of reference)	In a theoretically-frozen moment in time (one theoretical instant)
Where do facts exist? (inertial frame of reference)	In a theoretically-frozen position in space (one theoretical place)
How do we get facts? (reference experience)	By measuring something physical in a single theoretically-frozen place and time
Can we picture facts? (is there a visual reference?)	**Yes** (but only in the one theoretically-frozen place and time)
Are facts linear or fractal?	**Linear** (non linear things are averaged or ignored)
Do existing facts ever change?	**No** (although new measurements can always generate new facts)
With facts, how many selves do we have? (psychological reference)	We have **no self** (we have no sense of the mind or body—we are watching from somewhere outside of the mind and body; the state of neither body nor mind)
Examples:	The lamp cost $5.00. It stands 23" tall. It takes 3-way bulbs up to 250 watts.
Keywords:	Statistics, grades, theoretical *quantities* (as opposed to theoretical *qualities*), amounts; physically quantifiable data, things observed at a **now-line** (in a specific instant); linear states of being

What is a Fact?

(Facts are what the materialist wise man tells you is true.)

Facts—the First Great Truth

What is a fact? Let's start with some facts about facts. Facts are the materialist wise man's truth, and because there are only four wise men, a full twenty-five percent of all truths are based on facts.

Where do facts come from? They come from measuring physical things. And yes, we can and often do try to fool ourselves into believing we can measure things which are not physical—feelings and ideas, for instance. We can't. Neither is measurable in the true sense of the word *measure*. Nor can we measure stories, although as you'll find out later in the chapter, all stories contain references to physical measurements. The point is, facts are the only truth we can measure. Thus this quality—that we've measured something—is what makes a truth a fact.

This then is the key to understanding facts—the idea that all facts are *measurements*. What makes something a measurement? To see, we're going to use something I call, "the three core qualities of truth"—a reference time, a reference place, and a reference experience. Indeed, these three qualities are what allow us to define any and all things in our world, including the first of the four truths—facts. How? Let's see.

The Three Core Qualities of Facts

[The First Quality of Truth] All truths occur within a reference time frame. For facts, this reference time frame is *a theoretically-frozen instant—a single, standing-still moment in time.* In order to come up with a fact then, we must imagine that we've stopped time, and that in that imaginary frozen moment, we measure something as it crosses a "now-line." We can of course measure this thing at other times. But part of what makes a measurement a fact is that this particular measurement occurs in a theoretically-unique instant, while all other observations of this particular person, place, or thing will occur in other than this particular instant.

The point is, whenever we wish to refer to a fact, part of what we must refer to is to the single theoretically-frozen moment in time in which this measurement was taken, the moment in which it crossed a "now-line." Thus because all facts must occur in a single, frozen moment in time, a *single now-line moment* is one of the three things which make something a fact.

[The Second Quality of Truth] All truths occur in a reference place. For facts, this reference place is *a theoretically still, unchanging physical position*. Thus while other similar facts may occur in similar places, none can occur in this exact physical position.

Know that understanding what makes this true can take a bit of effort. Essentially, it's that all things physical are forever moving (e.g. the Earth, the stars, the Sun, our atoms). Moreover while we frequently refer to things as if they do stand still, in the real world, this cannot happen. All real world things are in constant motion. Thus change is what defines something as being in the real world.

This means no matter how carefully we remeasure something, in the time inbetween measurements, this thing moves through space. And because space and time are really two inextricable aspects of one and the same thing—spacetime—when we limit the time in which a fact exists to one theoretically-frozen instant, we simultaneously limit the physical position of this measurement to a single point in space.

Whenever we wish to refer to a fact then, part of what we must refer to is the theoretical still point in space wherein this measurement took place. Or stated more formally, the *theoretically-frozen position in space* in which this measurement occurred.

[The Third Quality of Truth] All truths describe a reference experience, some sort of meaningful mental or physical experience. With facts, we derive this reference experience from *measuring something physical in a single theoretically-frozen place and time*. Please note that because there are two ways in which we can make these measurements, there are two kinds of facts. The first kind we'll refer to as RSSs—References to a Standard Scale (e.g. your grade on the final math exam, your age, height, and weight). The second kind we'll refer to as ODEs—Observations of a Definite Event (e.g. the winner of a horse race, what you ate last night for dinner).

This then is the third part of what we must refer to when we wish to refer to a fact—an experience wherein we measure something, either an RSS or an ODE.

If we now combine these three qualities, we arrive at a clear and distinct way to define facts. Facts are the outcome of measuring something physical [1] in one theoretically-frozen time, [2] at one theoretically-frozen place, [3] with a single measurement event, either an RSS or an ODE.

The First Type of Facts—References to a Standard Scale

Now let's look more closely at the two ways we can measure things. In the first, we refer to a standard scale. In the second, we observe a definite event. We'll start with the easier of the two, References to a Standard Scale. What is a standard scale anyway?

A standard scale is any commonly accepted, numeric scale of measurement with which people describe the physical properties of some real world person, place, or thing. Lengths, widths, heights, and depths described in feet, inches, yards, miles, and kilometers. Measurements of sound, such as volume (in decibels), pitch (in hertz), and tempo (beats per minute). Sizes of containers described in ounces, quarts, liters, and gallons. Weights of things described in ounces, grams, pounds, and tons.

We also use standard scales to measure things like angles (in degrees), color (in angstroms), and temperature (in degrees F or C), as well as things like speed (in rpm, mph), price (in euros, dollars), clothing sizes (44R, size 10), and even menstrual periods (in days, twenty-eight last month, twenty-nine the month before).

So what is an RSS?

An RSS is a reference to a time wherein we used one of these standard scales to numerically count or measure some aspect of a physical thing. Twenty-four apples (*standard scale: counting numbers*). Twenty-four pound paper (*standard scale: pounds*). A twenty-four inch high rubber plant (*standard scale: inches*). A twenty-four year old, foxy lady (*standard scale: years*). Each of these measurements results in a fact. Each of these facts is an RSS. Moreover, in theory, we must do a lot of this kind of measuring, as about one out of every eight personal truths contain a reference to a standard scale.

The Second Type of Facts—Observed Definite Events

What about the second kind of facts—Observed Definite Events? What makes something an ODE?

Let's start by defining the phrase "definite event." A *definite event* is a reference to a commonly named, non-numeric physical world occurrence. A closing on a mortgage. The dinner you cooked last night. The flat tire you got last Saturday. The time you caught your cat peeing on your bed.

What is an ODE then? It's a reference to any single instance wherein we observe one of these non-numeric, physical occurrences. I closed on my mortgage in Nanuet on Tuesday. I cooked dinner for my girlfriend at home last night. Last Saturday, on my way home, I got a flat tire. I caught my cat peeing on my new lace bedspread this morning.

Can you find the three core qualities of truth for ODE facts in each of these events—one place, one time, and one definite event?

I closed on my mortgage (*one definite event*) in Nanuet (*one place*) on Tuesday (*one time*). I cooked dinner for my girlfriend (*one definite event*) at home (*one place*) last night (*one time*). Last Saturday (*one time*), on my way home (*one place*), I got a flat tire (*one definite event*). I caught my cat peeing (*one definite event*) on my new lace bedspread (*one place, thank God*) this morning (*one time, ditto*).

Did you also notice how these ODEs differ from the RSSs I mentioned a moment ago (e.g. twenty-four apples, twenty-four pound paper, a twenty-four inch high rubber plant, a twenty-four year old foxy lady)? With RSSs, we use a standard scale to numerically count and measure something. With ODEs, nothing is counted or numerically measured per se. We simply observe some commonly named event or state of being. For example, take the cat peeing on your bed. This observation—catching your cat peeing on your bed—is most certainly a definite event. We call it *definite* because we can precisely define it. No need for science here. We all know what this looks like. And we call it an *event* because it's so common, most people who have cats would recognize it as soon as you say it. (Maybe you should have gotten a dog?)

When exactly does this event become an ODE fact? In the moment in which you observe it occurring. A moment before, the day is going well. A moment later, the new bedspread is history. And in the time in-between these two moments, your cat goes from being your little darling to a royal pain in the ass. Moreover, whomever observes the little bugger doing this experiences an ODE fact.

RSSs and ODEs—Can You Tell the Difference Yet?

At this point, you might want to take a few minutes to try writing out some examples, say ten RSS facts followed by ten ODE facts. Can you do it? Great. If not, before moving on, it might be good to review what you've read so far.

To begin with, all facts are *measurements*, from the Greek word "metron," meaning *limited proportion*. Also, all facts occur in the same amount of theoretically-limited space and time, a single theoretically-frozen place and moment. The difference between these two kinds of facts then lies in how you make these measurements.

Did you use a standard scale? Or did you simply observe an event?

With RSS facts, you use a standard scale to numerically count and or measure the physical properties of something, the size of a blouse, say, or the height of a closet. With ODE facts, you use your powers of observation to note that some particular physical event has occurred, the dog barfing on the living room carpet or your seven year old knocking over the knock-off ming vase again.

Realize that when I say, we "note," I mean we "measure something with our eyes." This measurement may even include seeing an RSS fact, such as when you look at the size label in an article of clothing. To be considered an RSS though, you would need to be doing something like telling someone this number, as in, "Yes, Mildred, the blouse is a size 7." Referring to the size of a blouse is an RSS. Whereas to be an ODE, you would need to be doing something like making sure they had the blouse in your friend's size, as in, "Yes, Mildred, they have your size." Checking to see if a store has someone's size is an ODE.

Still confused? Don't worry. You'll catch on soon enough. And besides, you're far from the only one who has trouble identifying facts. As we're about to see, even professional fact gatherers, such as scientists and researchers, have their struggles.

Subjective Measurements Are Not Facts

A part of how we've defined facts is that they measure something physical. What about the kinds of measurements psychologists, social researchers, and political pollsters take—those we call subjective measurements? Don't these scales measure non physical things?

Indeed they do. At least, some people claim they do. In fact, these scales are purported to be able to "measure" all sorts of non physical stuff, from depression (*a feeling*) and creativity (*an idea*) to pain (*usually a feeling but sometimes an idea*) and satisfaction (*either a feeling or an idea, but not both*).

The thing is, while these imaginary scales do in some manner "measure" things, none of them result in tangible data, neither RSSs nor ODEs. At best these measurements roughly approximate people's opinions of things. Your cat's favorite food—most edible to left-in-the-bowl. Your husband's favorite brand of women's underwear—sexiest to scandalous. The importance of having a safe car—forty-two air bags should be mandatory to seat belts should be optional. And so on. And yes, these so-called measurements do have value and at times can guide our decisions. But there's nothing definite about these fuzzy outcomes. Thus they're opinions, not facts.

Problems occur only when we treat opinions as if they are hard facts. Conclusions based on these pseudo-facts inevitably lead to errors.

In the case of scientists and researchers, this can mean years of misguided efforts and dead ended research. And in the case of more mundane things like balancing a checkbook and managing credit card debt, this can lead to what in hindsight are some of our more questionable decisions.

Now before moving on to define our next truth, let's look at a few of the ways in which facts affect our lives.

A Few Interesting Ideas about Facts

In the next section, we're going to talk about stories and how, in their simplest incarnation, they derive from a series of ODE facts. In other words, ODE facts are the raw materials from which stories arise. Feelings and ideas may also, at times, refer to facts. However, only stories *must* contain facts.

Similarly, all lists derive entirely from facts. Each item on a list is either an RSS fact or an ODE fact. However, if a list has an overall order and intent, then this list is more than just a collection of facts. It is a story. For instance, while a phone book is a list of facts, a bus or train schedule is the story of where those trains or buses go for that period of time.

Then there's the way facts and intelligence go together, as in how being book smart refers to knowing facts. As opposed to having a high IQ which refers to knowing ideas (patterns). Having street smarts doesn't refer to knowing facts either. It refers to knowing stories (what's happening). As for how feelings and being smart go together, for the most part, we disregard this possibility. In some cases, we even see having feelings as not being smart. Of course, I have no facts to support this idea. Just my feelings.

Then we have the thing about how facts create tension. What I mean is, "knowing a fact is coming" is what creates the tension in everything from gambling and game shows to sex, sporting events, and action movies. Thus when the circus man is guessing a person's weight, it's an RSS fact that creates the tension. And when we're having sex and reaching for the big "O," it's an ODE fact that creates the tension. Either way, whenever we feel tension, it comes from waiting for a fact.

In addition, there's how facts can help or hurt us with overeating. You see, with overeating, you can have either facts or fat. The facts I'm referring to are things like, in this place and time, how many calories are on your plate? Or how many grams of fat are in this cupcake? Or how many Weight Watcher Points did I eat this morning? And so on. Knowing *why* these things matter can't make you thinner if you don't know the facts. Knowing *why* is the ideas. Knowing *how much* is the facts. And like I said, you can either have facts or fat. Measurements or mental masturbation. It's your choice. So chose wisely, grasshopper.

Similarly when people have problems being on time, not knowing the facts is the problem. Time-based commitments always derive from facts. This, in part, is why folks who struggle to be on time hate making appointments. Appointments—the fact of when you need to be somewhere—feel like traps to these folks. Are they trapped though? Not really. And in the real world, having an organized life can free your mind to do other things. Besides, no one says you have no say in how you schedule your appointments. So yes, in theory, committing to be somewhere on-time can feel like a trap. But being late is no picnic either.

The solution to being late, of course, in many ways parallels the solution I mentioned to overeating. You can either have facts, as in knowing when and where your next appointment is, or lateness—failures to be on time. To make this work though, you need to resolve yet another conflict the wise men create. Here, the idea of keeping one's options open (the advice of the rationalist wise man) directly conflicts with knowing the facts listed on a schedule (the advice of the materialist wise man). Don't be too mad at these guys for doing this though. They each have a point. And in truth, as I've been saying, to have a good life, we need to listen to all four of them. Really, we do.

Finally, a Story about Facts

I recently tried, in my office, to explain the four wise men to a client of mine. He then vehemently argued for that it was a fact that his wife was a bitch. I then tried to no avail to explain to him that his wife being a bitch is an idea. However, all attempts to explain why failed. In the end, I had to let it go. Moreover, having met his wife, he may be right.

It's still not a fact though.

Speaking of Feelings

Comedy is a feeling. Fact-based comedy is one of the three varieties of this feeling. In essence, fact-based comedy refers to sight gags and physical comedy in general. Examples of fact based comedians would be Robin Williams, Jerry Lewis, Jim Carrey, Norman Wisdom, Conan O'Brien, Mr. Bean, Lee Evans, Max Wall, Matthew Perry, Kathy Greenwood, The Three Stooges, and Lano & Woodley.

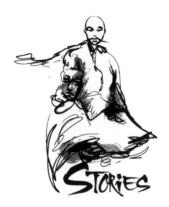

Stories

Where are stories true? (the horizontal axis position)	*Only* in the **real world** (stories are unknowable in theory)
In what time do stories exist? (temporal frame of reference)	In a single series of similarly-sized, consecutive times with an approximate beginning and end
Where do stories exist? (inertial frame of reference)	In a single series of similarly-sized, consecutive places which exist within a specific physical frame of reference
How do we get stories? (the reference experience)	By creating a cohesive series of similarly-sized, consecutive ODEs, all of which must occur within a single reference place and time with an approximate beginning and end
Can we picture stories? (is there a visual reference?)	**Yes** (except for changes between frames, which are invisible)
Are stories linear or fractal?	**Fractal** (may contain linear references)
Do existing stories ever change?	**Yes** (stories change each time they're told, even if only by emphasis)
With stories, how many selves do we have? (psychological reference)	We have **two physical selves** (we are both the narrator of our life and the one living this life—the state of only body, no mind)
First example:	I woke up, showered, ran downstairs, then fell. The light was off. It was dark.
Second example:	I saw the brown cat claw the couch, then I threw a ball at it, then it ran away.

What is a Story?

(Stories are what the empirical wise man tells you is true.)

The Second Great Truth—Stories

So what is a story? A story is a related sequence of three or more observed definite events. For instance—the black horse was out in front by a length *(first observed definite event)*, then the spotted horse pulled equal at the far turn *(second observed definite event)*, then the pale horse pulled ahead to win by a nose *(third observed definite event)*. Moreover, like facts, there are two kinds of stories—simple stories, like the one I just told, and complex stories. What's the difference?

The Two Types of Stories—Simple and Complex

A simple story is *a single sequence of at least three ODEs.* A complex story then inserts into this sequence feelings, extra facts, and or ideas. For example, to make our simple horse race story into a complex story, we might tell it something like this.

The black horse was out in front by a length *(observed definite event)*. Suddenly I felt physically ill *(feeling)*. I'd bet the rent on the darned spotted horse *(observed definite event)* and now it looked like he was falling asleep *(idea)*. But wait *(idea)*. The spotted horse, the one I'd bet on, just pulled ahead at the far turn *(observed definite event)*. Wow *(feeling)*. Maybe I will win after all *(idea)*. But as I continued to look through my field glasses, I saw the pale horse pull up even *(observed definite event)*.

Suddenly I realized *(feeling)* that the pale horse looked suspiciously like my ex-mother-in-law *(idea)*. Then, as the pale horse pulled ahead to win by a nose *(observed definite event)*, I realized that the old nag was my ex-mother-in-law *(observed definite event)*! With a jockey riding on her back *(observed definite event)*! Holy cow *(feeling)*. My horse, the spotted horse, just lost to my ex-mother-in-law *(observed definite event)*. I knew I should have shot the old bag when I had the chance *(idea)*.

Former mother-in-law jokes aside, the thing to notice here is how the heart and soul of both types of stories is a sequence of ODEs. And since ODEs are measurements, the key to understanding stories is to understand the phrase "consecutive measurements." What makes something a consecutive measurement? Let's find out.

The Three Core Qualities of Stories

Is this getting a bit complicated? It can seem like it at first. It's not really though, given you've learned what facts are.

How are stories different from facts? To see, we're going to look at how the three core qualities which define stories differ from those which define facts. In truth, learning to see these differences is a good way to tell the four truths apart. For instance, for facts we said the reference time was *one theoretical instant*, the reference place was *one theoretical fixed position*, and the reference experience was *one measurement*, either an RSS or an ODE. How are stories different?

[The First Quality of Truth] All truths occur within a reference time frame. For stories, this reference time frame is *a single sequence of similarly-sized times*. Here, by similarly-sized times, I mean the events in stories all need to occur at the same temporal scale. This scale can be anything from a series of sporting-event snapshots or a series of Paleolithic epochs to a sequence of chores done on a weekend or a sequence of careers in a lifetime. Each of these sequences contains a group of similarly-sized events. Thus each sequence meets the first criteria for stories—that the ODEs must occur in similar amounts of time.

In addition, to be considered a story, this entire sequence needs to occur within one specific time frame. In other words, a story must have a designated beginning and end. This differs markedly from facts which occur in a single theoretical instant. In effect, for facts, the beginning is the end, whereas with stories, the beginning and end are separate and different.

With respect to time then, to be considered a story, this story must refer to *a single series of similarly-sized, consecutive times with an approximate beginning and end*, whereas facts occur in a single theoretical instant.

[The Second Quality of Truth] All truths occur in a reference place. Unlike facts which occur in one unchanging physical position, stories can and often do refer to several physical locations. However, while the physical location within a story can change, the size of these changes must be similar. For instance, a simple story might be: I got out of bed, went downstairs, put on the coffee, jumped in the shower, then left for work. Here the physical location changed five times. However, all five changes were similar in size.

At the same time, while a story's location can change many times within a story, these changes must all occur within one reference place. Of course, this reference place, and the events occurring within it, can sometimes be quite large, even as large as our galaxy. And this is fine. To be a considered a story, though, the events must all occur within a single reference place—from Mars to Earth (reference place: our solar system), from Maine to New York (reference place: the northeastern USA), from office to home (reference place: your neighborhood), from the bedroom to the kitchen (reference place: your home), from your left eye to your right (reference place: your face).

Please realize this reference place can also be a non physical location as well. This works because we treat minds as if they exist in physical places. In addition, when we imagine stories, what we imagine includes the physical places in which these stories occur. Thus even imaginary stories can meet this second requirement.

With respect to a reference place then, to be considered a story, this story must include *a single series of references to similarly-sized, consecutive places which exist within a specific physical frame of reference.*

[The Third Quality of Truth] All truths describe a reference experience, some sort of meaningful mental or physical experience. With stories, the thing we must experience is *the overarching physical category of experience communicated by the story.* Having a cohesive physical similarity is what changes this series of facts into a story. Thus all stories must include some sort of cohesive theme. Moreover, while this theme must be communicated by a single sequence of at least three ODEs, any combination of ideas, extra facts, and feelings may be inserted into this sequence.

Please note there are many ways in which the four wise men may try to confuse you. For example, they may suggest that you insert yourself into the story, or guess the ending before it comes. They may also suggest you offer the story teller alternate endings, or seek hidden meanings, or make it a never-ending story, or suggest conflicting viewpoints. Indeed, these four wise-asses have an almost unending bag of tricks with which to obscure a story teller's theme. Fortunately we need not identify a story's theme in order to know it is a story. We need only know this theme exists, a category of physical experience upon which this sequence of events is based.

To sum it up then, a story is a cohesive series of at least three similarly-sized, consecutive ODEs, all of which must occur within a single reference place and time with an approximate beginning and end. Moreover, while you may insert into this story, extra facts, feelings, and ideas, none of these additions need exist.

Measured Glances as the Basis for Stories

At this point, it might be a good idea to talk a bit more about how we can measure ODE facts with our eyes. Yes, I did briefly mention this idea in the section on facts. However, being as ODEs are the basis of stories, I'd like to expand on this idea a bit.

What makes me say that ODEs are measurements? A clue lies in how often we allude to taking a measured glance at something. For instance, doing a quick search on the Internet for the phrase "measured glance" gleaned over 100,000 references. In effect, what we're referring to here is to how we sometimes measure things with our eyes—as opposed to a casual glance, wherein we simply give things a quick once over. With stories, of course, what we are looking for is recognizable non-numeric events. Thus these measured glances all result in ODEs.

Why bring this up? Because the heart and soul of every story is a series of these kinds of measured glances. To wit, consider these examples.

As I looked out the living room window, I saw my six year old Evel Knievel fall off his bike. Before I could start for the door, though, I saw he was up and fine. Or—When Ralph volunteered to tune my piano, I was glad. But as he bent over the piano, I noticed he had a bad case of plumber's butt. When did his ass get that big? I vowed right then and there that this would be our last date. Or—When that bitch, Rita, looked over at me, I tried to hold back the tears. But when she jejunely checked her watch and told me it was time for me to leave, I lost my composure and let her have it. Or—As Tim the Magnificent sat down on my couch, I caught him checking his wallet for a condom. So I reached behind the couch for my king-sized mace and set the nozzle on super stun.

All these stories consist of sequences of measured glances. All these measured glances are ODEs.

A Story about Having No Stories

There are also times wherein you can't come up with ODEs. For instance, when I was seven, I tried briefly to become a cub scout, the operative word being, "tried." I never was quite able to become one. Indeed, looking back, I remember this failed adventure quite well. In particular, I remember the day our little band of seven year olds arrived at the den mother's house too early, only to have her bulldog chase us up onto the roof of her car. This dreadful siege then continued for what seemed like ages until at last, Mike M. took my trombone out of its case and attacked the bulldog head on. At which point, the dog turned tail and ran. I guess the dog had yet to learn to appreciate classical music being played by a maniacal seven-year old.

Soon after that, the den mother came home. We then went inside and proceeded to do some cub scout stuff, including that she decided I would try to get the "telling a story" badge. Being as the wise man I trusted least back then was the empirical wise man, I couldn't think of a single thing to say. Then, after what seemed to be an even more painful succession of dread-filled minutes, a thoroughly-exasperated den mother said we could try another time.

Ironically, if I had to pick which wise man I trust most today, it would be the empirical wise man. I literally love telling stories. At the same time, whenever I witness someone struggling to find their words, it reminds me of the pain I felt that day.

The thing I'm pointing out of course is how the four wise men can blind us. I could have told the bulldog story. It didn't occur to me.

All Ideas Should Lead Back to Stories

In the next section, we'll be talking about how ideas emerge from stories. Something to keep in mind then is that the reverse is also true—that all ideas should lead back to stories. To see this in action, consider the idea of teaching stories.

What I mean is, for millennia, wise men have been using teaching stories to get their ideas across. Aesop's "The Tortoise and the Hare" fable. Jesus and his wedding wine parable. Plato's story of the shadows in the cave. Lincoln and his "I don't need a law" speech. At the same time, these same wise men have also often stirred people into action with the form of spoken ideas referred to as "slogans." Bill Wilson and A.A.'s "one day at a time." Christianity's "do unto others."

The thing to notice here is how tying a slogan back to a wise man's story deepens the meaning. For instance, take the Christian saying, "do unto others." In all likelihood, this slogan came out of a story in which Jesus reversed something first century b.c.e. rabbi, Hillel the Elder, said—"that which is hateful to you, do not do to your fellow. That is the whole Torah—the rest is explanation." And A.A. founder Bill Wilson may have derived the slogan "one day at a time" from the New Testament story in which Jesus said, "Take therefore no thought for the morrow: for the morrow shall take thought for the things of itself." (Mt. 6:34 KJV).

The point is, slogans sans stories are thin wisdoms, to say the least. Conversely, grounding ideas in stories breathes life, strength, and clarity into them.

Must These Stories Be True?

What happens if it turns out that the stories behind these slogans turn out to be false? Does this in any way negate the worth of these ideas?

As we'll see in the next section, behind every idea is a group of related stories. Thus even if the stories are fabricated, just being aware that an idea is rooted in stories can deepen our interest in this idea. At the same time, if these stories are filled with hate, then they will poison the idea. This said, the more you use stories to ground your ideas, the better the chances your idea will be understood. Indeed, were you to ask yourself, each time you encountered a new idea, if you knew the story behind it, you'd not only improve your chances to learn this idea. You'd significantly better your chances to find personal truth.

How Stories Reveal the Good in Religion

Speaking of stories and religious slogans, an idea Karl Marx is said to have coined is that religion is the "opium of the masses." I, myself, think religion can be a wonderful thing, especially if it teaches us how to love each other more. Sadly, more times than not, the opposite is the case. Religions teach us to hate. At the same time, despite the compensatory hatred some folks, including Karl, throw back in religion's direction, none of this hatred is the fault of religion per se. Rather, it stems mainly from the part of human nature which to me, is the real "opium of the masses." Blame.

To wit, we live in an age where being able to instantly connect to each other is a high priority. In part, this is because we all like telling stories. Unfortunately, the more we become able to do this, the more we blame. Indeed, blaming people has now become an international pastime. Talk about throwing people to the lions. Moreover, this blame includes not only the kind some religious folks heap on non believers. It also includes the kind those wishing to scapegoat religion toss back in religion's direction.

Ironically, the remedy for all this blame, like most truth, lies hidden in plain sight—revisit the stories of the founders of these religions. There you'll often find the true intention of this religion—practice tolerance, love your fellow wise man, and find your personal truth.

Do Stories Prevent Enlightenment?

One of the rationalist wise man's favorite ideas is that our goal in life should be to become enlightened, and that to do this we need to boil our ideas down to their essence—no stories allowed. In other words, to the rationalist wise man, only pure ideas can lead to happiness. Stories just clutter up life.

So is this true? Will ignoring stories lead to a better life? To be honest, I've seen better advice written on the inside of men's room stalls. To aspire to become a mind dissociated from the warm, messy roundness of a real life is to aspire to being other than human. Maybe after I die, this will appeal to me. Right now, I kind of like being human, messy roundness and all.

The point? One thing that makes us human is that we tend to tell stories. This is why those among us who are most in touch with their humanity—our children, for instance—so love hearing stories. Seen in this way, I think becoming enlightened is sort of like aspiring to become a tasteless, colorless, odorless ball of light. Thus while to some, this kind of sterilized existence may sound appealing, to me, living without stories sounds more like eating cardboard for a living. It might pay well, but would you really want to do it?

Stories Are Best Told One at a Time

Finally, there is the idea that many times, what we call stories—things like O'Henry's short story, *The Last Leaf,* for instance—are, by the present definition, not one story, but rather several stories within a story. Thus when we refer to whole books and movies as "stories," we're more referring to the idea that there is an overarching theme which runs throughout the entire work than to that this book or movie meets the criteria for being a "story." In reality then, these books and movies are not stories. Rather, they're groups of stories under the umbrella of one idea. Thus if you want to get the story straight, try to keep in mind that whenever you tell a story, this is best done one story at a time.

Feelings about Stories

As I've said previously, comedy is a feeling, and stories are one of the three forms this feeling takes. In comedy, the basic story is a sitcom. The Punch and Judy shows of sixteenth century England are an early example. However, included in what this wise man thinks is funny are acts like Laurel and Hardy, TV shows like The Honeymooners and Saturday Night Live, and movies like Animal House. Also the comedians Jonathan Winters, Paula Poundstone, Paul Merton, Tony Slattery, Josie Lawrence, Jim Sweeney, Steve Steen, Wayne Brady, Ryan Stiles, Colin Mochrie, Drew Carey, Greg Proops, John Sessions, Neil Mullarkey, Kathy Greenwood.

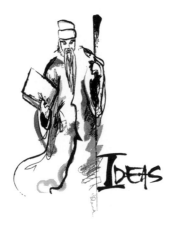

Where are ideas true? (the horizontal axis position)	*Only* **in theory** (ideas are unknowable in the real world)
In what time do ideas exist? (temporal frame of reference)	**In all now-line moments** (ideas exist simultaneously in all times)
Where do ideas exist? (inertial frame of reference)	**In all places** (ideas exist simultaneously in all places)
How do we get ideas? (the reference experience)	By verbally condensing the mental and or physical aspects of what our mind observes in a set of stories into an overarching meaning or meanings
Can we picture ideas? (is there a visual reference?)	**No** (mental states cannot be pictured)
Are ideas linear or fractal?	**Linear** (but they may refer to fractals)
Do existing ideas ever change?	**No** (but they can lead to new ideas)
With ideas, how many selves do we have? (psychological reference)	We have **two mental selves** (we are both the thinker and the one watching the thinker—the state of only mind, no body)
Examples:	Lamps light rooms. Rooms get dark. Darkness is the absence of light.
Keywords:	Understandings, meanings, cause and effect logic, theoretical *qualities* (as opposed to theoretical *quantities*), idealized states of being, induction, deduction, inferences

What is an Idea?

(Ideas are what the rationalist wise man tells you is true.)

The Third Great Truth—Ideas

Now we come to the third great truth, the first of the mental wisdoms. Know that in many ways, this makes this truth hard to describe. Why? Because there is no way to picture a mental truth, as it isn't physical. For instance, take the idea of time. I'm sure you can picture sitting for an hour in a doctor's waiting room. But can you picture the hour itself? Of course, not. Hours are an idea. Similarly, the idea of childhood. Certainly, you can picture events from your childhood, a birthday party, for instance, or being in the school play. But can you picture childhood itself? Again, no. Childhood is an idea.

This, then, is the first thing to know about ideas. Because they are mental not physical, we cannot picture them. And yes, we can and often do picture something physical when we think about an idea. But if you do picture something when you think of an idea, the thing you're picturing is never the idea itself. Rather, it's something which, to you, physically represents this idea, usually something drawn from a story wherein this idea is the story's central theme.

Are you having trouble seeing what I'm saying here? Then consider the idea of a hole. Yes, it's easy to picture something with a hole in it, say, a moth eaten, beige cashmere sweater. But because holes are not something physical but rather, the absence of something physical, no one can picture the holes themselves. Holes are an idea.

How about the idea of shapes, for example, the idea of a square? Certainly you can picture trying to fit a square blue peg into a round orange hole. But can you picture the actual square? Not sure what I'm getting at here? Well think about it. We define a square as a shape having four equal sides and four equal angles. But nowhere in this definition do we mention anything physical—the colors or lines, for instance. So when you think you are picturing a square in your mind, the square blue peg, for instance, what are you picturing? Obviously, it's isn't the *idea* of the square. Ideas aren't physical. Thus as Plato alluded to, a square blue peg is merely an imperfect replica of a square and not the idea itself.

Why don't we realize we can't picture ideas? Say hello to the beloved wise men again—they've been baffling us with this one for years. Ironically, even this idea—that ideas can't be pictured, can't be pictured. Which explains why ideas can be so hard to learn. Ideas are invisible.

At the same time, if you know about the two physical world wise men, this all falls into place. Ground your ideas in facts and stories and they come to life. We'll talk more about this later.

The Two Types of Ideas—Natural and Supernatural

The next thing to know about ideas is that they come in two flavors, *natural ideas* and *supernatural ideas*. Here, natural ideas stem from the generalizations we make about the physical things we observe in sets of related stories, whereas supernatural ideas arise out of the generalizations we make about the logical causes for, motives behind, judgments about, and psychological effects of what we refer to in natural ideas.

Said very simply, natural ideas are generalizations we make which describe how real world things exist or change. The idea of seasons— summer, for instance, or the condition of alcoholism—late or early stage, or the concept of right angles—approaching or separating, or the state of your physical health—improving or deteriorating. Supernatural ideas then come from the generalizations we make about our natural ideas, such as that summers are hot and nasty, that alcoholism can or can't be cured, that well-built walls need to always meet at right angles, or that eating the right foods can make you healthy.

To sum it up then, natural ideas are ideas about stories, while supernatural ideas are ideas about ideas, and both are rooted in the generalizations we make after observing groups of similar stories.

Time to Test Yourself—Writing Out Some Examples

Now it's time to see if you've understood what I just said. To do this, try writing out ten natural ideas. Then try writing out ten supernatural ideas which might derive from these ten natural ideas. If at first it feels a bit tough, don't give up. You'll get it if you persist.

For example, two natural ideas which you might write down are that horses win races and that people watch horse races. Both these generalizations come entirely from physical observations of things you see in a group of horse race stories. Some supernatural ideas which might then arise from these two natural ideas would be that horse races attract pathological gamblers. Or that gambling on horses is addictive. Or that jockeys mistreat horses. Or that it's wrong to race horses.

Are you having trouble seeing the difference? Then try focusing on the word *natural*. Now ask yourself if your ideas describe something about the physical nature of the things you've referred to. For instance, *oak leaves contain chlorophyll* generalizes an aspect of the physical nature of oak leaves. As does *commercial airplanes have wings* about airplanes, and *text books have pages* about books, and *cell phones have ring tones* about cell phones.

Now remember that supernatural ideas come from the generalizations we make about the logical causes for, motives behind, judgments about, and the psychological effects of what we refer to in natural ideas. For instance, "your neighbors fertilized their lawn with horse manure mixed with oak leaves so you would stop traipsing across their lawn" assumes something about your neighbor's motives. And, "most airlines deny it, but to save money, they skimp on wing safety features" makes a judgment about airline economics. Or, "rich kids who deface their text book pages cause school taxes to increase disproportionately in wealthier school districts" posits a logical cause for the tax increase. And, "teenagers deliberately alter their parent's cell phone ring tones to confuse their parents" makes a judgment about teenagers and ring tones.

Finally, if you took this last idea and played with it a bit, you could just as easily end up with the other three forms of supernatural ideas. *Teenagers deliberately install cell phone ring tones which annoy their parents so they will leave them alone* makes an assumption about motive. *Giving teenagers cell phones which they can modify increases movie theater disturbances* infers a logical cause for movie theater disturbances. *The ring tone of an average teenager's cell phone disturbs most adults* posits a psychological effect.

Here again, the key to discerning between the two kinds of ideas lies in remembering that the word *natural* refers to the physical properties of something. Does what you're referring to refer to something physical? Then it's a natural idea—an idea about a story. However if your idea refers to the logical cause for, motive behind, a judgment about, or the psychological effect of what you saw, then it's a supernatural idea—an idea about an idea.

The Three Core Qualities of Ideas

Now let's look at the third great truth—ideas—through the filter of the three core qualities—time, place, and experience. How do the core qualities of ideas differ from those which define stories. Remember, for stories the reference time frame is a single series of similarly-sized, consecutive now moments with an approximate beginning and end, the reference place is a single series of similarly-sized, consecutive places existing within a specific inertial frame of reference, and the reference experience is the overarching mental and or physical category of experience communicated by how these times and places change. How are ideas different?

[The First Quality of Truth] All truths occur within a reference time frame. For ideas, this reference time frame is *all now-line moments*. For instance, the idea that "horses win races" has neither a beginning nor an end. Thus, this idea will be true forever—it exists in all times.

Of course, what allows us to say this is that we're talking about a theoretical truth and not something which physically exists. In other words, while, in the real world, there may be a time wherein there will be no more horse races, still, the idea that horses can win races would not end, not even then. In theory, horses will always be able win races, even if there are no more horses. Thus unlike the two real world truths which can exist only in limited amounts of time, because ideas exist in theory, they exist forever. This makes the reference time frame for ideas *all now-line moments*.

[The Second Quality of Truth] All truths occur in a reference place. With ideas, because they are a theoretical truth, they have no physical limitations. Thus the reference place for ideas is *all places*, everywhere.

How can this be? Consider the idea that lamps light rooms. All lamps can theoretically light all rooms. This says nothing about when can they light these rooms or how well they can do this. Only that they can.

So where do these rooms exist? In theory, they can exist anywhere and everywhere. Similarly, where can horses race? Again, in theory, anywhere and everywhere. Thus while both physical world truths—facts and stories—can exist only in limited places, ideas can exist anywhere and everywhere. This makes the reference place for ideas *all places*.

[The Third Quality of Truth] All truths describe a reference experience, some sort of meaningful mental or physical experience. From a mind body perspective, ideas refer to the mental process of the mind expressing in words what the mind has observed in groups of stories. Please note that to the mind, the actual physical aspects of the things we've observed are seen as something to subtract out. As such, these physical aspects are seen as anything from unimportant and inconsequential to an intrusion on the idea-deriving process. Moreover, this need to purify our ideas by deleting all physical references from them makes describing the reference experience for ideas rather difficult. Know we'll address this difficulty a bit later. For now, the thing to know is that, for ideas, the reference experience is the mind talking in words about what it observes in a category of stories.

Or to voice this more in the language of ideas, to have an idea, we must be *verbally condensing the mental and or physical aspects of what our mind observes in a set of stories into an overarching meaning or meanings.*

Putting these three core qualities together then, we can define an idea as an experience true in all places and in all times, wherein the mind expresses in words abstract generalizations about what it has seen in a category of stories, either about the natural aspects of what it has seen in these stories, or about the ideas it has expressed about what it has seen in these stories.

Why the Rationalist Wise Man Loves Technical Language

Has my use of the terms *natural* and *supernatural* confused you? To be honest, I'd be surprised if it hasn't. Both words carry a lot of baggage, so much in fact that I spent a long time considering whether to use them or not. In the end, given my sense of what I'm trying to express here, the rationalist wise man convinced me that these two terms fit best. The thing is, by choosing to go ahead and accept his advice, I must now face something I would have preferred to put off until later in the book—the idea that the words we use often do more to obscure the truth than to clarify it.

Take, for example, one of the rationalist wise man's favorite things— the idea that some words have more than one meaning. The words *natural* and *supernatural* certainly do. This can lead different dictionaries to prioritize these meanings differently, making the problem even worse. Oh, does he like it when that happens. Add to this that we tend to interpret words rather than to take them literally and we can end up with quite a mess. Which is why we often spend great amounts of time arguing the meanings of words versus what we meant to say.

So what's the best way for us to handle this? First and foremost, there is the idea that what we picture when we hear words determines what these words mean to us. We'll discuss how we can benefit from knowing this in a moment. Before we do, let's talk a bit about a somewhat less common problem—how people tend to misunderstand technical words which are also used as ordinary words.

Take the two words I've just used, *natural* and *supernatural*. Because I've based some of my technical language on these two ordinary words, I've heightened the risk you'll misconstrue what I'm saying. At the same time, to ask you to learn two new words could make things even more complicated. Who wants to do that anyway? It's a pain in the ass to learn new words. (Shut up, "R.")

So what do we do? It's simple, actually. Dictionaries of technical words have a special name. They're called *glossaries*. Moreover, were you to look up the origin of this word, you'd find it comes from a Greek word meaning "tongues" or "languages." I mention this because you can use this knowledge to dramatically improve your ability to understand technical words. All you need to do is to treat these words as if they are vocabulary from a foreign language. And yes, remembering to do this can be a bit of a challenge, especially when you already know an ordinary meaning for the word. However, if you do remember to do this, you'll learn far more, including from this series of books.

How Pictures Give Ideas Their Meaning

Now let's look at how the pictures words provoke in our minds determine what these words mean to us. Why would this matter? Because as I said at the beginning of the section, things like holes, squares, childhood, and hours aren't physical. Thus, we cannot picture them. What we can picture of course are the stories from which we draw these ideas. Moreover, since the words we use to express our ideas stem directly from these physical examples, the more examples you can picture, the better you'll understand your ideas.

For instance, say we're talking about the idea of holes. What's the first thing this word brings to mind? A natural idea, like the holes in swiss cheese, or a supernatural idea, like the holes in people's arguments?

Now notice what happens when I add two more pictures, a second natural example—the holes in a screen door screen, and a second supernatural example—the holes in people's heads.

Here, we see a good example of how adding pictures to an idea deepens our understanding of this idea. We also see how grouping these pictures together can sometimes lead to a new idea, as in the obvious point we can draw from this example—that it's easier to picture natural ideas (ideas about physical things) than supernatural ideas (ideas about ideas).

Is any of this making sense to you? It should. The idea here is simple. Your ability to grasp the meaning of an idea rests largely on your ability to picture examples. This in part is what makes it so difficult to understand technical words. Because technical words, by design, refer to specific techniques, often, we have no stories from which to draw our examples.

This said, my main point is that to understand an idea, you must be able to picture physical examples. The more, the better. This is what underlies the writer's maxim, "show, don't tell," as in, show examples rather than tell ideas. Moreover, the success of anything involving ideas depends largely on the quality of the examples we use. Learning, teaching, communicating in general—all require good, solid, real world examples.

How Wounds Keep Us From Picturing Ideas

Speaking of learning, do you realize your ability to learn depends mainly on your ability to picture words? In essence, to learn an idea, you must be able to find good pictures for this idea. Equally important is being aware of those times wherein you can't find a picture, as this means you've encountered a blind spot. Moreover, until you heal this blind spot, your ability to learn this idea will be limited to logic and parroting other people's truths.

What exactly does this inability to picture an example mean about your ability to learn? For instance, does it mean that you're just bad at picturing this particular subject? To see, you'll need to investigate further, by seeking out additional examples. Moreover, this makes sense. In theory, we can picture even simple words in a great many ways. So without a group of similar pictures to contrast and compare, how can you know for sure which of these meanings is the right one?

This in part is what may have motivated Noam Chomsky to say that language is a "discrete infinity." In other words, despite it's theoretically knowable structure, in the real world, language varies infinitely. And yes, there may be times wherein you correctly guess the meaning of an idea without a visual example. But is this how you want to live—basing your personal truth on guesses?

In truth, we all have times wherein we cannot picture a word, even when given an example. Here, the problem lies not with language per se, nor with intelligence. Rather, it lies with something I mentioned back in chapter one—the idea that if you're startled while you're saying or hearing a word, that this can permanently program your mind to go blank each time you think of this word. This causes you to become unable to picture this word, even if you can logically understand it. And when this happens, try as you may, you'll be unable to picture even obvious examples.

Reservations aside as to the nature of startles, are you beginning to see how being unable to picture an idea affects your ability to grasp its meaning? To begin with, let me say this. Going blank when you hear or read words is the root of most misunderstandings, including most "you never listen to me" complaints. It's also the problem underlying most difficulties with learning in general, including everything from not retaining what you read and struggling to remain present in classrooms to thinking you're bad at math and not being able to take good notes.

This also explains why trying harder in classrooms fails most times. Trying harder to do something you cannot picture only sets people up for failure. And leads to more feelings of hopelessness.

Can you see yet why I'm saying that picturing ideas is so important? Again, it's because what we picture determines what our ideas mean to us. Thus if we can't picture examples, we have no way to know what an idea means. This, indeed, may be the most counter-intuitive thing to know about ideas—*that ideas have no inherent meanings*. And yes, the stories you draw your ideas from may include non visual content, such as logic and reasoning. If asked, this logic may allow you to recant what seem like good understandings. These words may even sound beautifully lyrical or logically astute. But without visual content to flesh out your logic, your ideas will more resemble uncolored outlines in a child's coloring book than ideas with clear and distinct meanings.

Testing Yourself by Trying to Picture Some Words

Are you finding this concept—that we must picture words—difficult to accept? Admittedly, it's not how we're normally taught to process words. Fortunately, it's easy enough to learn though. After all, it's simple. You can either picture a word or you can't.

Still not clear? Then try this. Try picturing the word *truth*. Can you do it? Good. Now go ask someone else to picture this word as well. Then compare notes. Know that one or both of you may be unable to picture examples for this word. But if you both can, you'll be surprised at how dissimilar your pictures will be.

What if you can't find a picture for the word *truth*? What then?

First take a big breath. Then make a note of this word. You might even want to do this for the entire series of books—write down the words you find hard to grasp. Know that in Book III, I'm going to ask you to make a list of words you can't picture, so you can try your hand at healing some of your wounds. Wounds aside though, let's try another word.

This time try picturing the word *supernatural*. What do you picture when you hear this word? An alien scene from the X Files? Ghosts chasing you around a haunted house? Madame Zola answering her psychic hotline? Bo Derek's breasts as she runs on the beach?

The thing to notice of course is how what you're picturing affects this word's meaning. Obviously there's a big difference between the apparently supernatural movements of Bo Derek's magnificent mammaries and calling

1-800 dial-a-psychic. At least, I hope there is. Then again, maybe you're thinking of calling a psychic to get the 411 on bouncing mammaries?

Are you getting this? No? Okay. Then let's try one more example. This time try picturing the word *love*. What comes to mind when you think of this word? Can you picture anything at all? If you can, take a moment to jot down what you see, along with what it means to you.

Now go call five close friends and ask them to do this as well. And yes, they may think you're crazy for asking them to do this, but what the heck. You only live once. Or twice. Or more, depending on whom you ask these days. Whatever the case, go call them, then write down what they picture. Now set this paper aside, as we're going to come back to it in a moment.

Me? What did I picture? My first picture was a scene in which a four year old boy is laughing as he tumbles on a lawn in summer amidst a dozen beagle puppies. My next picture was a thirteen year old girl being handed a single red rose by a tall gangly, fourteen year old, zit-faced boy. My next picture was an elderly couple at the Jersey shore. They're sitting side by side on a weathered bench, wrinkly faces smiling and age-spotted hands gently holding each other. Next I pictured a tan, muscular lifeguard in choppy water, arm around the body of a frightened forty-two year old waitress who just almost drowned while on her first vacation in nine years.

Did you too see more than one picture? If so, did you notice how your sense of the word *love* changed as your pictures changed? Moreover, it's not hard to see why. Obviously there are big differences between a four year old boy laughing, a thirteen year old girl smiling, an elderly couple still in love, and a lifeguard saving a life. The point is, your pictures determine what your ideas mean to you. Thus the more pictures you have for your ideas, the deeper your understandings will be.

For Others to Understand Us, We Must Have Similar Pictures

Now go get the paper I had you write a moment ago and take a few minutes to review it. Did any of your pictures resemble mine? How about yours and your friends' pictures? Did any of your pictures match any of theirs? In all likelihood, few, if any of your pictures will have matched anyone else's. So let me ask you. How do you think these differences have been affecting your ability to communicate with others, including with your close friends?

Finally let's try one more example. This time imagine you and one of your close friends are talking about joining an online dating site, and that she has just asked you what kind of person you're looking to meet.

Rich, tall, dark, handsome, and sensitive, right? The thing is, each of these ideas can be pictured in a myriad of ways, and if you doubt me, just ask this friend what she pictures when you say rich, tall, dark, handsome, and sensitive. Are we talking the rich Corinthian leather tan of a muscled aristocrat from southern France? Or are we talking the astonishingly glossy, blue-black skin of a wealthy, cat-bodied Ethiopian industrialist? And can you even picture aristocrats or industrialists who are sensitive?

Are you beginning to see the extent to which pictures affect your ability to understand ideas? And how, the more you pay attention to what you're picturing, the more you'll understand? In reality, I cannot emphasize this idea enough—that *your truth is what you picture.* This means, if you pay more attention to what you're picturing, you'll breathe new life into all your relationships. Or, if you choose to ignore this advice, you can expect your relationships to grow stale over time. Again, it's your choice. So choose wisely, grasshopper.

If You Change Your Pictures, Your Ideas Change Too

A few moments ago, when I pictured the word *love*, I had several pictures come up. So what happens to us when this occurs in real life— during the course of a conversation, say, or when we visually digress to a parallel story? In truth, all people digress during conversations. It may even be fun at times. But if we fail to notice our pictures changing, we'll have quite a hard time staying focused.

Taking this idea a step further, do you realize that many people use this concept to improve their lives. For instance, take creative visualization. Creative visualization is based on the idea that if you change what you picture, you change your life. Olympic coaches use this idea when they train their athletes to picture success. Also, noticing what you picture is the sine qua non of most meditation practices. In addition, many motivational speakers use this same concept, telling people vividly-painful stories which turn-out surprisingly well. And as you'll find out in chapter ten, when people unexpectedly picture a good outcome, the meaning of their suffering permanently changes for the better.

How about you? Would you like to see for yourself how the third great truth can dramatically improve your life? It's simple. Spend ten minutes a day, each day, for the next thirty days, working with words which feel important to you. Take your time and try to pick words which have an especially powerful meaning to you. For instance, on the first day, you might write down the word *spiritual,* or the word *courage,* or the word *healing.* Then sit quietly somewhere, for the next five minutes, while you picture this word. Then, when you're done, next to this word, write down the pictures it brought to mind.

Along with this, each day, try asking some friends what they picture when they hear these words, then write down what they see as well.

Finally, take some time to compare pictures with them. I promise you'll be stunned by the many differences. As well as by how this exercise brings the two of you closer. You may even experience some of those surprise endings I mentioned a moment ago. Perhaps they'll even change your life. At the every least though, you'll know more about yourself and your friends, all this from a few minutes spent picturing words.

Misusing the Word *Idea* to Mean an Estimate

A less common problem people face when they can't picture an idea is that they try to feign understanding with the phrase, "Yes, I have an idea of what you're saying." Here, the phrase *I have an idea* refers to having the gist of something. Since ideas get their meanings from pictures though, this simply can't be true. You can't have the gist of a picture. You either can see something or you can't.

What these folks would be better off saying of course is, "I haven't a freakin' clue what this idea means!" Or perhaps they could just ask for clarification, preferably by asking for a few examples. The thing is, most folks don't like admitting that they didn't understand an idea. And you can't blame them. The world tends to be rather rough on those who struggle to learn. Sometimes, downright cruel.

The point is, when we use the word *idea* to mean that we get the *gist* of what's being said, we do this because we're unable to picture it. When this happens, it can mean only one thing—that we have yet to find a personal truth for this idea. Thus anyone who claims to be getting the gist of something is talking out of their sun-don't-shine place.

Not the best place for a personal truth to emerge from.

How False Stories Create Impersonal Truths

Yet one more thing to know about ideas is that only true stories lead to true ideas. For instance, take the idea of *separate but equal* which permeated laws in the US from 1896 until 1954 and pragmatic practice from the end of the civil war (1865) until almost the end of the twentieth century. In part, this idea was based on a distortion of Darwin's theories called "Social Darwinism"—the idea that some races are inherently inferior. This led to the belief that African Americans, among others, were biologically inferior and could be treated as such with no harm done.

Sadly, many stories, all false, were concocted to support this idea. Then in 1947, the husband and wife team of Clark and Clark developed a simple way to test for whether this belief was harming children. This test involved a set of four plastic, black and white, diaper-clad dolls, identical except for color. These dolls were just ordinary toys that cost 50 cents each at the Woolworth's on 125th Street in Harlem.

The Clarks showed these dolls to black children between the ages of three and seven, then asked them questions to determine racial perception and preference. Almost all the children readily identified the race of the dolls. But when asked to choose which dolls were nice—which they would like to play with—and which were a nice color—many of these children chose the white dolls, whereas when asked which dolls looked bad, many of the children chose the black dolls.

In a second study (1950), the Clarks gave children outline drawings of a boy and girl and asked them to color the figures the same color as themselves. Many of the children with dark complexions colored the figures with a white or yellow crayon. The Clarks concluded that "prejudice, discrimination, and segregation" caused black children to develop a sense of inferiority and self-hatred. And in 1954, the US Supreme Court agreed and ruled accordingly.

To Have Personal Truth, You Must Have Your Own Experiences

The story I've just told you derives in part from the Library of Congress exhibition, *With An Even Hand, Brown Versus Board of Education at Fifty*. This exhibit describes the idea of these tests pretty well. However, if you'd like to get a better sense of what this idea truly means, try picturing two plastic, diaper-clad white dolls and two plastic, diaper-clad black dolls laid out on a desk in front of you. Now picture yourself standing to the side of this desk some six or so feet away.

Now imagine a little black, six year old girl sitting at this desk, with me sitting across from her. Now picture me asking this child the actual questions the children were asked in 1947.

(1) Give me the doll that you want to play with.
(she picks the white doll).
(2) Give me the doll that is a nice doll.
(she picks the white doll).
(3) Give me the doll that looks bad.
(she picks the black doll).

(4) Give me the doll that is a nice color.
   (she picks the white doll).
(5) Give me the doll that looks like a white child.
   (she picks the white doll).
(6) Give me the doll that looks like a colored child.
   (she picks the black doll).
(7) Give me the doll that looks like a Negro child.
   (she picks the black doll).
(8) Give me the doll that looks like you.
   (she picks the white doll).

Imagine this six year old girl picking the white doll when asked questions 1, 2, 4, and 8. Stories like this were what led to the Supreme Court ruling that *separate but equal* was unconstitutional.

Now let me ask you. Do you think things have changed much since then? Well if you do, then you might be surprised by what teen filmmaker Kiri Davis found. In 2005, she recreated the Clark's study in a seven minute film titled *A Girl Like Me*. To her shock, her results were similar to what the Clarks found in the late 1940s and early 1950s. Fifteen out of the twenty-one children preferred the lighter doll when asked to choose "the nice doll." Moreover, despite Davis' obvious lack of scientific rigour, the point still stands. Being treated differently can lead to self hate.

Keep in mind the point I've been making here—that only true stories lead to true ideas, while false stories only lead to false ideas. Moreover, when it comes to self hate, obviously, this feeling can never be based on true ideas. For this truth about self hate to help us though, we must know which stories are true and which are not. This means, based on the amount of skin-color prejudice still around, false stories must still abound. Hopefully this book will help this to happen less.

Feelings about Ideas

Big breath now. This may feel like a jarring transition. Nothing I've just told you is funny. Even so, before we close this section, I need to remind you that comedy is a feeling, and that ideas are one of the three sources for this feeling, the other two being facts and stories.

Examples of idea-based comedy would be the word play of Mark Twain, Groucho Marx, Lenny Bruce, Johnny Carson, William Shakespeare, The Simpsons, Oscar Wilde, Woody Allen, and George Carlin, as well as the satire of Dennis Miller, David Letterman, and Jay Leno.

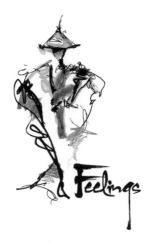

Where are feelings true? (the horizontal axis position)	*Only* in **the real world** (feelings are unknowable in theory)
In what time do feelings exist? (temporal frame of reference)	Feelings have no reference time (the experience of **timelessness**)
Where do feelings exist? (inertial frame of reference)	Feelings have no reference place (the experience of **placelessness**)
How do we get feelings? (the reference experience)	From experiencing something which exceeds our ability to describe with facts, stories, and ideas
Can we picture feelings? (is there a visual reference?)	**No** (mental states cannot be pictured)
Are feelings linear or fractal?	**Fractal** (nonlinear)
Do existing feelings ever change?	**Yes** (constantly, in the observer's mind)
With feelings, how many selves do we have? (psychological reference)	We have **one holistic self** (the state wherein the mind and body are connected and in sync, we are simultaneously watching from both the mind and the body)
Examples:	I'm sad, angry, distressed, confused; I feel like I'm bad (I broke the lamp)
Keywords:	emotions, intuition, spiritual sensations, passive verbs, pain; what exceeds your capacity to put into words

What is a Feeling?

(Feelings are what the spiritual wise man tells you is true.)

The Fourth Great Truth—Feelings

Finally, we come to the most difficult truth of all to define. Why? Because, like ideas, feelings are mental. Thus we cannot picture them. Also, the word *feelings*, like many words, can mean many things. Touch, intuition, emotion, sensation—which one is it? It's hard to say.

The real problem with defining feelings, however, is none of these things. The real problem is that when we ask people what they're feeling, this request shuts their feelings off. This in part explains why most of us hate being asked this question. As soon as we're asked, our feelings evaporate, leaving us with nothing to say.

This is also why subjectively measuring feelings does not lead to facts. You can't measure something that doesn't stand still. And yes, people's answers may agree, time and time again. These answers may also make logical sense. But if what you're measuring ceases to exist the minute you measure it, then you can't very well consider these answers valid.

This then is the first thing to know about feelings. There is no way to test for them, let alone be sure they exist. Thus while you can, on occasion, empathically connect and by doing so, gain insight into what people feel, this is not a measurement either, as the same limitations apply.

How then can we hope to define the fourth great truth? The only way I know is to say this. Feelings are what you experience when you try to access the immeasurable. You experience feelings whenever something exceeds your capacity for words. Moreover, the more this experience exceeds your capacity for words, the stronger your feelings become. Until, at last, they exceed your body's ability to contain. At which point, you cry, scream, smile, laugh, or groan.

Does this inability to find words *cause* your feelings?

Not really, albeit you can have feelings about this inability. Rather, being unable to find the words to express something creates a sort of spiritual "black hole" in you, and when you try to determine what's in this hole, this effort creates your feelings. No surprise then that these spiritual black holes often occur at pivotal moments during important conversations. And when this happens, you can so lose your words that you zone out and just go blank.

You can also feel feelings, then lose touch with them, by uttering words mindlessly. When people sob, or when they drink too much, this happens a lot. To look at these folks, you would think that feelings were pouring out of them. But the word *feel* implies awareness, and mindlessly uttered sounds do not qualify.

How can we know for sure that we're aware of our feelings? At the risk of confusing you, we need words to be sure. At the same time, because facts, stories, and ideas act like an off-switch for feelings, if these words express an idea, fact, or story, then these words shut your feelings off.

This then is the second thing to know about feelings. Feelings involve words being used in a special way—in two ways at once, actually. One, the failure to find the words for something is what creates the container for our feelings—the hole. Two, in order to be aware of these feelings, we must find the words to express this failure.

How can something be both "beyond words" and "voiced with words?" Admittedly this description must sound confusing. Then again, that's the point. If we can discern feelings only by exceeding our capacity to describe something in words, then feeling the inadequacy of this definition as we consider it implies we are on the right track. Intuitively this feels right, does it not? Trying to experience this definition feels a lot like what it is trying to define?

At the same time, I am all too aware that this definition will leave most folks feeling unsatisfied. So what can we do to better define the fourth great truth?

A moment ago, I said that facts, stories, and ideas act like an off-switch for feelings, and herein lies the key. As it turns out, if we can learn to see this off-switch in action, we can get a good sense of what feelings are. Before I show you how to do this though, I first need to discuss a more essential aspect of feelings—the idea that there are two types of feelings, *mind feelings* and *body feelings*. And yes, I'm well aware that to some, this division—mind versus body, may sound dubious at best. It's not really. But before the rationalist wise man convinces you otherwise, allow me to explain what I mean by these two phrases.

The Two Types of Feelings—Mind and Body

If you've read the summary pages at the beginning of each section, you've noticed that a part of how I've defined each of the four great truths is with our sense of how this truth affects our sense of self—either through our sense of mind, or body, or both. Why haven't I mentioned this in the prior three sections? Mainly because I'm saving the full blown mind body discussion for chapter four. I've also been able to define the prior three truths without having to refer to the mind and body. However, with feelings, I cannot do this, as changes in our sense of self are one of the few things we can definitively state about feelings.

What kinds of changes am I referring to? There are many analogies we could use. For instance, say we are talking about a country that has two provinces, a northern province and a southern province. If we likened ourselves to this country, we might call mind feelings the northern province and body feelings the southern province. One country. Two provinces. Or say we liken ourselves to a building with two floors. We could call mind feelings the upper floor and body feelings the lower floor. One building. Two floors. Or say we liken ourselves to the way time passes. We could call mind feelings the light of day and body feelings the dark of night. One diurnal cycle. Two time units. Or say we liken ourselves to the universe itself. We could call mind feelings the heavens and body feelings the earth. One universe. Two dimensions.

Now try to picture what it would feel like for you to move between these pairs of opposites. Can you sense how these movements would affect your feelings? You'd likely feel quite differently in the northern and southern provinces of a country, and on the upper and lower floors of a building, and during the day versus at night. As for the spiritual concept of heaven and earth, even here, you'd likely feel quite differently, given you could get a feel for what these two states might be like.

How Ancient Symbols Represent the Two Kinds of Feelings

Speaking of how it feels to move between pairs of opposites, did you know that many ancient spiritual traditions include symbols which portray this aspect of feelings. Take, for example, the Celtic cross of pre-Christian northern Europe. Here, the cross represents all things physical (the body), and the circle, the hole in the physical world from which all things spiritual emerge (the mind). Similarly, the Egyptian ankh, another circle / cross combination. Here we see a closed loop (the mind) above a tau cross (the body). Ancient Egyptians believed this symbolized "the key to understanding life." And a third example would be the Tao symbol of China—the Tai Chi Tu, considered by some to symbolize the essential nature of our world. In this case, we see a transverse wave dividing a circle into two halves, with the white half representing the mind and the heavens, the black half, the body and the earth, and the circle, the hole or abyss from which this pair of opposites emerge.

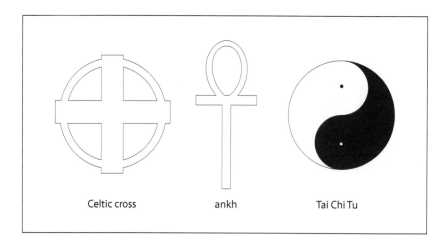

Celtic cross   ankh   Tai Chi Tu

In each of these symbols, we see represented the nature of change in our world, including the idea that this nature is rooted in what we feel when we change between a pair of complementary opposites. Philosophers call this pair of opposites, a *duality*. My point for telling you this?

These changes between pairs of opposites are where feelings come from. They come from those times wherein we see the coin flip, so to speak. In other words, life events, in and of themselves, do not cause feelings. Like ideas, life events have no inherent meanings. At least, until we experience a personally meaningful change during these life events.

This is why you felt your sense of self change when you imagined my examples. When you move between a pair of opposites, your sense of self changes, and this change generates your feelings.

Why does this happen? Because we too are dual in nature. Each of us is one person sensing life from two personal perspectives—from the mind and from the body. Moreover, the basis of this dual perspective is that this gives us two ways to sense change. First, we can sense change with our body. Second, we can sense it with our mind. And whenever we shift between these two sources of sensation, we experience feelings.

The Surprising Origin of the Tao Symbol—Facts

Feeling a bit uneasy with where this discussion has been going? If so, then remember this. It's the spiritual wise man's truth we're discussing here. His truth is never factual, or logical. Thus, if this discussion seems hard to swallow, it's likely your trusted wise man is either the materialist wise man or the rationalist wise man. Both of them are always claiming that anything the spiritual wise man says is nonsense. If this is you, then allow me to ground what I've been saying in some science. Did you know, for instance, that the Tao symbol derives from facts gathered similarly to how modern science gathers facts? And that it was these facts which led to the philosophical and spiritual practices which Taoists teach today?

Where did these facts come from?

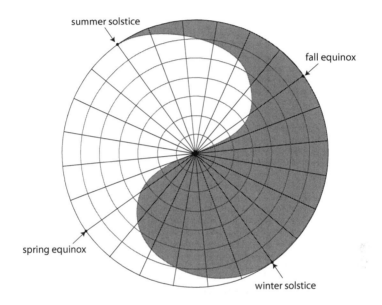

Imagine you are a monk living in southern China some two plus thousand years ago. In the center of your monastery is a courtyard, and in the center of this courtyard is a large white, circular stone patio with a 4" hole in the center. In this hole stands an 8 foot high pole, and each day you place a stone on this patio to mark the midday sun's shadow as it gets blocked by this pole. Of course, some days would be cloudy or overcast. Thus on those days, there would be no measurable shadow. More times than not though, there would be one. And because the position of the sun changes over the course of the year, by placing stones on this patio, a shadow shape would gradually emerge.

What would you see if you were to do this? If you lived anywhere near 23° northern latitude, you would see the origin of the Tao symbol—a circle which contains an unmarked white yang on left, and a shadowy black yin on the right.

What does this drawing have to teach us about feelings? To show you, I'm going to ask you to picture a large glass sphere. Now imagine holding this sphere in your hands and inside it, there are two colored smokes, one black and one white. Now imagine these two smokes are flowing toward each other, the white smoke chasing the black, and the black smoke chasing the white. Moreover, while it seems they each keep turning into the other, neither grows smaller in size.

Were you able to do it? If so, did you feel anything? To be honest, it's hard to do. If you stay with it though, you'll begin to feel things, including that you'll feel drawn into what you see. This happens because whenever we picture movement, our mind and body connect. In effect, our two sources of feelings temporarily function as two end points on a continuum. This causes us to momentarily lose touch with the duality which permeates our world, including that we cease to feel separate from what we're picturing. And when this happens, we can literally feel like we have stepped into the scene.

Realize this change in our sense of self is the essence of all genuine spiritual experiences. Here you lose your sense of separateness and merge into what you see. This is also why some spiritual practices call this state "selflessness," and why philosophers call the state wherein two complementary opposites merge, a *unity*.

The Master Continuum of Feelings

This brings us to the third thing we can say about feelings. If we juxtapose this unity with the feeling of duality we felt before, we can now define the master continuum on which all feelings exist. This continuum ranges from the experiences wherein we feel profoundly alone and separate from all things—because our mind and body feel separate—to the experiences wherein we feel profoundly connected to and at one with all things—because our mind and body feel like one and the same.

In a moment, we'll begin to explore the duality end of this continuum, as we look at what makes mind feelings differ from body feelings. Before we do, and at the risk of provoking more skepticism, I want you to know we'll be returning to this continuum, and to the spiritual symbols which represent it, many times throughout the book.

Still think these symbols are just the spiritual wise man's hooey? Then you should know that no less than Nobel prize winning physicist, Niels Bohr, made one of them—the Tao symbol, the central feature in his family crest in 1947. Why? He said it represented one of his contributions to theoretical physics—the principle of *complementarity*—the idea that nothing in physics can be defined without defining it's opposite. We'll talk about this idea in depth in a later chapter.

As for what makes mind feelings different from body feelings, let's see if I can frustrate you any more than I already have.

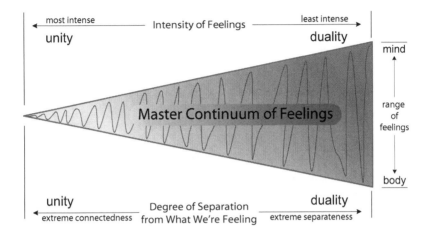

Why Feelings Provoke Mind Body Questions

In the previous two subsections, we spoke about the roles unity and duality play in feelings. Essentially, I explained that personally experiencing changes between pairs of opposites is what causes our feelings. In the next two subsections, we're going to look at how these feelings often impair our ability to make decisions. This happens because we feel pressured to choose between what feels true to our mind and what feels true to our body. This then creates an ambivalence in us that can make it hard to know what's truth.

Of course, most times, we don't notice this pressure, let alone call these feelings, mind body choices. But if you picture the following situations, I suspect you'll find the questions they pose familiar. Ready?

When you feel tired as you get up in the morning, what is this? Is this a body feeling, as in you feel unrested and groggy? Or is this a mind feeling, as in your head has been busy all night and now needs a rest? And when you feel foolish and embarrassed, what it this? Is this the physically yucky feeling that floods into you after someone tells you, during the school play, that your fly is open? Or is this the deafening mental blankness you feel when your science teacher calls on you in class and you can't come up with an answer?

How about people who say they love walking on beaches late at night. Are they feeling body feelings, as in they love the smell of salty breezes and the sounds of breaking ocean waves? Or are they feeling mind feelings, as in they feel nearer to God when they're this close to nature? And what about when your grandfather says he's got a hunch that it's going to rain. Is he feeling a body feeling, as in his joints are aching? Or is he feeling a mind feeling, as in he's intuitively sensing the statistical probability it will rain?

In each of these situations, we see the potential to experience a life situation in two ways, either as a mind oriented experience or as a body oriented experience. Not sure why this matters? Well think about it. Say you've been feeling kind of down lately. Depressed even. What kind of therapy would you seek? A physical therapy, such as what your psychiatrist, Dr. Feelgood might prescribe? Or a mental therapy, such as what your talk therapist, Ms. Compassionate Understanding, might engage in? Or say one of your neighbors has been blasting their stereo in the middle of the night. What would you more likely do? Seek a physical remedy, such as calling the police, hoping they shoot the bastard? Or a mental remedy, such as calling your lawyer, Barrister Sidney Vicious?

How about if you were focusing on your health. How would you go about it? Would you concentrate on your physical health, by eating better, taking vitamins, and enrolling at Sam Goldenbody's Gym? Or would you concentrate on your mental health, by taking a class in Akkadian philosophy and enrolling in Venus Astralplane's meditation and self exploration group? And what about if you were considering a job offer. Would you focus more on the physical aspects of the job, such as on the salary, hours, travel, and ergonomic desk and chair? Or would you focus more on the mental aspects of the job, as in the low levels of stress, intellectual challenge, and chance to be involved in decisions such as where Ms. Partedlegs sits?

Mind Feelings or Body Feelings—How Do We Decide?

Attempts at humor aside, my point here is simple. Regardless of whether you realize it or not, each time you experience feelings, you face a decision—is this feeling coming from your mind or your body? This decision then biases your solutions toward either your mind or body. And yes, most times you won't realize you are categorizing your problems. Or your solutions. You may not even believe a mind body distinction exists. Yet even from these few examples, it's easy to see, each time you experience feelings, you'll feel urges to decide where they're coming from.

Still having trouble seeing this? Let's try a few more situations. See if you agree with my answers.

Say you have a broken toe. This feeling originates in your body, right? Whereas if you have a broken heart, these feelings originate in your mind, yes? And what about your mixed-up sense of smell. These feelings come from your body, right? Whereas your mixed-up sense of loyalty comes from your mind? Yes?

So how do we decide which it is? This one is easy to see. For the most part, we base our decisions on whether we can see, or logically identify, a physical point of origin. If we can, then we assume these feelings originate in the body and require a physical solution. If not, we assume they're coming from the mind and require a mental solution.

Let's try a few more examples. Say, for instance, you banged your thumb with a hammer, or stuck yourself with a pin. In both cases, if asked, you'd likely point to the site of the physical injury as the origin of what you were feeling. If, however, you were feeling hammered by heartache, or stuck in a difficult decision, then you'd likely classify these feelings as mind feelings, as they have no apparent physical origin point.

This then is how we decide where our feelings are coming from. First we look for a physical origin point and if we find one, we see these feelings as body feelings. If we find no physical origin point, however, then we see these feelings as mind feelings. And yes, most people will not use the words *mind* and *body* in their answers. However, if asked—or if what they're experiencing feels important enough—they'll definitely feel urges to ask these kinds of questions, even without knowing why.

All Feelings Simultaneously Affect the Mind and Body

What I've just said is that each time we experience feelings, we feel urges to decide where they are coming from—whether from the body or from the mind. The thing is, if we pay close attention, we find that feelings always occur in both places simultaneously. Think a thought and it will affect your body. Feel your body and it will affect your thoughts.

Don't believe me? This one is easy enough to test for. Tap on the back of your left hand with a pen or pencil and try to have no thoughts while remaining physically aware of this tapping. Or taste a slice of pizza and try to remain mentally aware you're eating while becoming physically unaware. Yes, you can detach from both these situations if you let yourself zone out. But even zoning out affects both your mind and body.

What makes us believe otherwise?

The simple truth is, it's the wise men at it again, undermining our sense of reality. Here, the materialist and empirical wise men convince us that we should trust only what we can see. Hence our bias toward seeing physical origin points as the source of our feelings.

This belief also leads us to consider a wide variety of curious proposals. For example, I've read a lot lately about that if pills can change our feelings, then this proves feelings must be brain-chemical based. And that if evolution exists, then Darwinian survival-mechanisms must be the author of our feelings about God and the divine.

Of course, most materialists who promote these kinds of ideas seem to disregard the obvious counterpoints, e.g. that if feelings were only brain-chemical based, then there could be no placebo effect, and that if God were nothing more than a survival instinct, then no religion would promote self sacrifice and do-unto-others. Then again, before you put all the blame on the materialist wise man, you should know it's not all his fault either.

For instance, were you to listen to the empirical wise man's stories about spirituality, you'd realize there are just as many folks who hold the opposing view—that the body is temporary and disposable and that the mind / soul / spirit is the only permanent reality. As for these folks, I'm not sure how they'd feel about donating their bodies to science this afternoon. But I'd be willing to bet, if asked, we'd see some world class back-pedaling.

Wise men's obfuscations aside, my point is, despite our tendencies to divide our life experiences into body-based and mind-based experiences, if pushed, we find a second reality—the mind body unity. Moreover, while it's the duality of mind and body which underlies our sense that we have two types of feelings, it's the mind-body unity that gives this truth its name—spiritual truth. We'll talk about why in a moment. Before we do, let's sum up what we have said so far.

Summing Up the Two Types of Feelings—Mind and Body

The spiritual wise man's truth exists because we live in a world filled with pairs of opposites, a state philosophers call *duality*. Feelings are the way we human beings experience shifts within this duality.

In addition, because we, by nature, are ourselves a part of this duality, our feelings seem to have two points of origin. This causes us to experience feelings in two ways—either separately, as a mind body duality, or collectively, as a mind body unity. Normally we feel the mind body duality. When we do, this creates an uncomfortable ambivalence in us which we try to resolve by seeking a physical origin point for our feelings.

If we find one, we say our feelings are coming from our body and our ambivalence is resolved. But if we don't, then we resolve this ambivalence by saying that our feelings are coming from our mind.

The thing is, if we pay close attention to what we're experiencing in these moments, we find that our feelings arise simultaneously in both our body and mind. Albeit, whenever we picture movement, a third option arises. In these situations, we lose touch with our sense of duality and merge into what we see. This leads some folks to conclude that the separation we normally feel, both internally and externally, is more perception than reality. So is it? Let's see.

Our Four Identities—the Four Versions of the Self

What we've just gone through covers most of the theory behind feelings—the impersonal stuff. Now we're going to explore why, in real life, this truth feels so personal. To wit, most times, when people reveal their feelings, we see this as them being personal. Moreover, because feelings involve the whole person—mind and body—this makes sense.

The problem is, we also use the word *feelings* to refer to "impersonal" experiences, such as when someone dispassionately recalls how she felt her friend's husband was wrong as usual (an opinion; an idea), or when a news reporter dispassionately reports, "witnesses felt sure the mailman bit the dog first" (either a story, or a fact). Here, the way these folks use the word *felt* makes it seem like they experienced feelings. However, saying they *felt* ideas, facts, and stories doesn't make these experiences, feelings.

What's causing the confusion? The other three wise men are disguising their truths as feelings. To do this, they're using one of the most argued, misunderstood, and difficult to describe concepts in all of psychology—the one psychologists refer to as the "self." Moreover, because what I'm about to tell you is largely based on my recent discoveries about the mind and body, it's likely to be quite different from what you've previously heard.

How different is it? To begin with, there have been many systems in which the self has played a part. For instance, in Carl Jung's system, there is one self. Here, Jung sees the self as an archetype which signifies the coherent whole, a unity of the conscious and unconscious parts of a person. In Heinz Kohut's system, there are two selves, a narcissistic self, and an idealized parental imago. And although Freudians might disagree, in Sigmund Freud's system, there are three "selves"—the "it" (the *id*), the "me" (the *ego*), and the "above me" (the *superego*).

How many selves do the wise men say there are?

The Four Views of the Self

The Spiritual Wise Man's Self

The Universal Self
(there is one self;
mind and body are connected)

Mind on

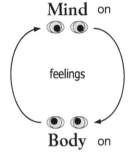

feelings

Body on

The Rationalist Wise Man's Self

The Thinking Self
(there are two selves;
mind is both, body doesn't exist)

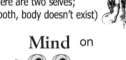

Mind on

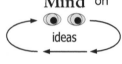

ideas

Body off

The Empirical Wise Man's Self

The Narrating Self
(there are two selves;
body is both, mind doesn't exist)

Mind off

stories

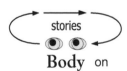

Body on

The Materialist Wise Man's Self

The Neutral Self
(there is no self;
neither mind nor body exist)

Mind off

facts

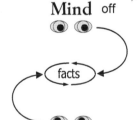

Body off

Surprisingly, just one, albeit, each wise man has his own way of seeing this self. In the materialist wise man's version of the self, we lose our identity. In the empirical and rationalist wise men's versions of the self, we have two identities, one watching the other. And in the spiritual wise man's version of the self, we have a single identity.

This then is the thing to pay close attention to as we go through these four versions of the self—how many identities make up each self. In the first version, we have one self with no identity. In the second and third, we have one self with two identities. And in the fourth, we have one self with one identity.

Now let's look in more detail at these four versions of the self.

The Materialist Wise Man's Version of the Self

Let's start with the first self, the one wherein we have no identity. This is how the materialist wise man sees life. To him, being part of what we observe contaminates the measurement. Thus, his advice to us is to stay out of the picture entirely.

What is it like to do this? To be honest, it feels strange. We know something has been observed—and that someone has made this observation. But try as we may, we cannot personally connect to this observation. This causes us to experience this truth like the legendary "neutral observer." Hence the name of this self—the *neutral self.*

What's it like to be in this state? Try looking into a mirror. Now look into your eyes and ask yourself who this person is. Most people, when they do this, feel strangely separate from the person they see in the mirror, as if this person is someone else. So who is the person in the mirror? Mentally, it's obvious. It's you. But personally, it's not obvious at all. Moreover, despite the logic that tells you that this image is you, the harder you try to connect to this person, the more separate you feel.

Having trouble getting what I'm saying? Then try this. Try recalling the first time you heard a recording of your voice, such as on an answering machine message. Do you remember how odd this felt? You knew the voice was yours, but it felt like someone else's. So whose voice was this, and who was hearing this voice? Again, while it was logically obvious, it still felt like someone else's voice.

This then is the materialist wise man's version of the self, the self you experience whenever you gather facts. In this state of being, you feel like you're looking down on life from some higher plane. It's as if you have become a ghost self, so separate and apart from what you're observing that you no longer have an identity. Hence this self—the *neutral self*, is the most impersonal of all. With this self, you no longer feel like a person.

The Empirical Wise Man's Version of the Self

Now let's look at how the empirical wise man says we should see the self. According to him, truth is visible only when we experience life as two identities—as a "subjective" identity, and as an "objective" identity. Here, by *subjective identity*, I mean the part of us who is observing a truth from outside of it, and by *objective identity*, I mean the part of us who is experiencing this truth from inside of it.

Please know, most folks have a hard time personally experiencing these two terms, and this is not surprising. They are, after all, both supernatural ideas. To understand them, then, you'll need to flesh out their logical meanings with visual examples. And to do this, we'll need to turn to our mirror story again. Only this time, you'll need to imagine you are telling me a story about a time when you were looking at yourself in a mirror.

So where are these two identities?

Your subjective self is the "you" who is telling me this story, and your objective self is the "you" who is looking into the mirror. In other words, the subject is the person telling the story, and the object is the person in the story.

The problem, of course, lies in the way we're using the word *object*. Referring to people as objects sounds cold and impersonal. And yes, whomever came up with this should probably be shot. However, if you think of the phrase, "the object of our desire," you'll realize, it's not so cold after all.

Unfortunately, semantics aren't the only problem here. You see, while the phrase "objective identity" always refers to the part of us in the picture, sometimes we create this "person" by projecting ourselves into an object. Here, examples would be velveteen rabbits (good old fluffy), exotic race cars (good old number 49), futuristic space ships (the good old battlestar Galactica), and beloved planets (good old mother Earth).

Something to keep in mind then about your objective identity is that, while this phrase always refers to a person, sometimes this "person" really is an object into which you've projected yourself.

Are you ready to tear your hair out? Know you're not alone. Even the more psychologically minded can find this concept difficult at best. I myself don't care much for calling these two identities, the subjective identity and the objective identity. However, since we've been using these terms for a long time now, I am choosing to honor this tradition. Moreover, if you keep in mind the empirical wise man's version of the mirror story, you'll do fine. Your subjective identity is the one telling the story. Your objective identity is the one looking into the mirror.

This then is the way the empirical wise man sees life. In this version of the self, we become the *narrating self*—the teller of stories. Here, we have two identities, one identity outside the story, the other, inside it. Moreover, while both identities play active roles in this version of the self, only one, the subjective identity, is actively narrating, while the other, the objective identity, acts only as an actor within the story.

Finally, because both these identities are bodies not minds, we feel *only* the physical aspects of this truth personally, while at the same time, we remain somewhat detached from the mental aspects of this truth.

The Rationalist Wise Man's Version of the Self

Now let's explore the rationalist wise man's version of the self. Here again, our self has two identities, a subjective identity and an objective identity. This time though, these two identities are both minds rather than bodies. And to see what this means, we'll need to adapt our mirror story to the rationalist wise man's style. Here, your subjective identity becomes the "you" whom is thinking about what your objective identity—the you who is looking into the mirror—is thinking.

Did you follow all that? I didn't think so. So let me try this again, this time, reversing the order while pointing out that both identities are thinkers. Here, the one thinking *in* the story is the objective identity, and the one thinking *about* this thinker is the subjective self.

Complicated, isn't it. In truth, it's really not. And if you plug this self into the answering machine story, you'll see why. To wit, in the Rationalist's version of the answering machine story, we are a mind imagining what we thought as we listened to our voice play back on an answering machine. Hence, our objective identity is the person who is thinking about what he is hearing, while our subjective self is the person who is thinking about what the person in the story is thinking.

Whew! Did you get all of it this time? Maybe it's harder than I thought. Whatever the case, don't give up. If you keep at it, you'll get it. Moreover, if you keep in mind what this self is called, it may help. It's called our *thinking self*. And similar to our *narrating self*, one identity exists within the story and one is watching from outside of the story.

Finally, because both identities are minds not bodies, we feel *only* the mental aspects of this truth personally, while we remain somewhat detached from the physical aspects of this truth. Which makes me think that perhaps I should be calling these last two truths, half-personal truths? Better yet, maybe you should just shoot me now.

The Spiritual Wise Man's Version of the Self

Finally we arrive at what most people find to be the easiest self to understand. This is the spiritual wise man's point of view—what it feels like to be a self. Here our subjective identity and our objective merge into one identity, making our identity identical to our self. Which is probably why many folks prefer to call this state of being, "being ourselves."

How would this self play out in our mirror story? Like all things felt, it's hard to put into words. Basically, we would have to add a second mirror to our story, this one behind us and visible in the first mirror. And if you've ever done this, you know how beautiful this can look—smaller and smaller mirrors all of which contain images of us in mirrors. Indeed, if you keep looking deeper and deeper into this scene, at some point, you'll feel like you've entered this mirror world.

Is this scene too hard to imagine? Then perhaps a better example would be to imagine you are standing on the edge of the Grand Canyon. Now imagine that as you look out at all this beauty, something about the scale of it begins to overwhelm you. You realize it's simply too much to take in. It's literally beyond words. And as you continue looking, you begin to feel like you're being drawn into the scene. Indeed, you may even reach the point wherein you suddenly feel that there's nothing to keep you from falling, yet another reaction to the mind and body merging—placelessness.

This then is the key to understanding the spiritual wise man's version of the self—noticing the way we lose all sense where we are—both internally; between our mind and body—and externally; between ourselves and the outside world. In this view, because our mind and body cease to be separate, we cease to perceive ourselves as being separate from the world. And according to the spiritual wise man, this is the truth. Separation is merely an illusion.

The thing to remember of course is that there are three other valid selves, and in each of those other selves we do feel separation. But because the spiritual wise man's self feels no separation, it's the mirror image to the materialist wise man's self. Thus, while the ghost identity of facts make them feel like the most impersonal truth, the unified identity of feelings makes them feel like the most personal truth.

Why Do Feelings Feel So Personal?

Why put you through so much brain-twisting, psychological stuff? Because this concept—having a self—explains why feelings are the only truth we can experience personally. In essence, it's the separation which prevents us from experiencing a truth personally. If we sense separation, then we feel things impersonally. If we sense no separation, then we experience things personally.

Why do we experience this separation, including that our mind and body feel separate? To be honest, we'll spend most of chapter four on this topic. At the same time, I need to at least briefly address this now.

The reason we experience separation is that, similar to the way energy moves more quickly than matter, sensations move through minds more quickly than through bodies. We also each have a comfort zone with regard to how quickly we process life. Those who speed through life prefer the quicker medium; the mind, whereas those who like a slower pace prefer the slower medium; the body. In both cases, this results in a time lag between our mind and body, and between us and life. And it's this time lag which causes us to feel separate, either from part of ourselves or from the rest of the world. Part of us literally feels like we're lagging behind.

Where does this time lag get inserted? With facts, we feel a time lag between what we're measuring and our whole self. This makes us perceive our mind and body as lagging behind the rest of the world. With stories we feel like our mind and all immaterial things lag behind our body. With ideas we feel like our body and all material things lag behind our mind. And with feelings, because the mind and body are in sync, there is no time lag.

Do you get the implications here? If one part of our self lags behind the other, we perceive ourselves as being out of sync, either with part of ourselves or with life. So why doesn't this happen when we experience feelings? Because whenever we experience feelings, we become unable to sense time. This causes any and all time lags to temporarily disappear, and while they're gone, our mind and body merge into one self.

This is what happens to us when we merge into mirrors within mirrors, or into the great natural beauty of the Grand Canyon. We cease to experience the time lag. Thus, we feel no sense of separation. In essence, our mind and body—and our sense of the world—all sync up. Hence the personal nature of feelings—we feel connected to our world.

A Clarification as to How I'm Using the Word *Personal*

Now before the more rational among you snag me on what may seem like an error, I need to elaborate on something—the way I've been using the word *personal* to refer to the self. The thing is, my stated purpose for this book is to teach you to find your *personal* truth. But I've just told you that we feel all feelings *personally*. So, by this, do I mean that my intention is to teach you to know your feelings?

In part, this is my intension. Feelings are one of the four great truths. However, I've also repeatedly told you that to be considered a personal truth, this truth must include all four wise men.

How can both things be true then? Start with this.

Back in chapter one, I defined personal truth as what emerges in us when we and all four wise men agree on something. By definition then, our personal truth involves all four wise men, plus a commonality which emerges in us. At the same time, because separation is what causes us to experience things impersonally—and because we experience no separation with feelings—we cannot experience feelings without feeling them personally. Hence my statement that all feelings feel personal.

So is this just a bunch of double-talk? Actually not. It only goes to show, yet again, how far these four masters of the sleight of mind and body will go to mix us up. You see, there is a big difference between defining something as a "personal truth" and feeling something "personally." My definition for personal truth is an idea. Feeling something personally is a feeling. Same root word. Two different wise men. Moreover, the experience of personal truth is far more than both these things put together. Rather, when we experience a personal truth, we change inside. Permanently.

In a way then, when we experience a personal truth, we experience something a lot more personal than feelings. We literally—in some way—become a new person. Thus despite the idea that personal truth and feelings have a lot in common, they're not the same. Yet another one of those hard-to-put-into words things about feelings.

The Three Core Qualities of Feelings

Now let's look at the three core qualities which define feelings, and at how they differ from those which define ideas. Remember, with ideas, the representative time frame is *all now moments;* forever and always— the reference place is *all places;* the entire universe—and the reference experience is one wherein *the mind expresses in words abstract generalizations about what it has seen in stories, either about the natural aspects of what it has seen in these stories, or about the ideas it has expressed about what it has seen in these stories.*

How are feelings different?

[The First Quality of Truth] All truths occur within a reference time frame. But with feelings, we cannot experience this reference. We can't experience time. This is why, if you're asked how long you've felt a feeling, you cannot come up with an answer. For example, if you fall in love and one moment later, ask yourself how long you've loved this person, you may know all too well that this love just began. Yet you will feel like you have loved this person forever. Moreover, if someone then asks you to pinpoint when this love began, you'll find yourself unable to do this as well. The point is, because we lose our sense of time when we feel feelings, we cannot place feelings in the field of time. Thus the reference time frame for feelings is *timelessness*—the experience of being outside of the field of time.

[The Second Quality of Truth] All truths occur in a reference place. However, for feelings, we can't describe this reference place. No descriptions seem true to us. Indeed, the more you try to describe this place, the more confused you feel. Are your feelings coming from inside you? From outside you? From your mind? From somewhere else? Frequently we say we know. But if we dig deeper, we find we cannot say.

At times then, you may feel your feelings are coming from your gut, such as when you're in the wrong part of town at the wrong time of day. Or you may feel like you're swimming in feelings, or drowning in them even, such as when you get fired unexpectedly or suddenly get asked for a divorce. In each of these cases, you can point to a physical location wherein the event occurred. But with respect to a reference place from whence your feelings are coming, you can tell neither where they are coming from nor where they are going to. Thus, for feelings, the reference place is *placelessness*—the experience of being outside the field of space.

[The Third Quality of Truth] All truths describe a reference experience, some sort of meaningful mental or physical experience. With feelings, the reference experience is being unable to find the words to describe what is happening to you. Thus, from an intellectual perspective, we could say that the mind and body are so busy observing each other that they lose their ability to voice the experience. However, while this description hints at what it's like to have feelings, in truth, it's but a mere shadow of the real experience.

So what is the reference experience for feelings? To be honest, like everything else we can point to about feelings, there is no way to put this experience into words, other than to say this. Feelings are what happen to us when something feels important, but this something exceeds our capacity to describe. Literally, the experience is beyond words.

Unfortunately, this is pretty much all we can say when it comes to the reference experience for feelings. Thus this reference experience suffers from the same problem that the reference time and place suffer from. All three are indescribable and cannot be put into words.

This leaves us with yet another totally inadequate, but absolutely accurate, conclusion. That the reference experience for feelings is that of *having something happen which exceeds our ability to describe.*

To sum this up then, feelings are defined as the timeless, placeless experience of having something personally important happen which exceeds our capacity to describe—an experience beyond words.

The Special Relationship Between Words and Feelings

In a moment we'll dig a bit deeper into the nature of feelings. Before we do, I first need to expand on what I said previously about how words play two roles in feelings. A moment ago, I said that the reference experience for feelings was having something exceed our ability to put into words. But in the introduction to this chapter, I referred to words being used with feelings, as in saying you hate to get up in the morning. So which is it? Must we be beyond words—or must we use "feelings" words?

The answer? As I said, it's both. And to see why, recall what I said about where feelings occur—they occur in the mind and body simultaneously. This means, if you're saying nothing—or if you're thinking no words—then your mind is contributing nothing. Likewise, if you're saying words, such as that "I'm sad," but your body is silent, where's your body's contribution?

At this point, perhaps a story might help. This story involves the game I'll introduce you to at the end of this book. To wit, I once played a wise men's game with my friend John, the friend I mentioned in chapter one. In it, he explored his decision to have his deaf two-year-old son get cochlear implants. The whole time we played, he cried from his entire body. Yet when we were done, he had no cards on the spiritual wise man. No feelings cards. When I then asked him to comment on what he saw, he right away acknowledged he had no feelings cards. Yet when I asked him why, he said, what difference would it make to tell me his feelings. "What would that change?"

Obviously, John's blind wise man is the spiritual wise man. Yet his whole body cried during this game. My point? Don't assume someone is feeling just because you see the signs of feelings in their body. To be considered feelings, a truth must be voiced both from the mind and the body. Tears without words are not sad feelings. Neither are sad words without watery eyes.

Using Words as Spiritual Expressions

But if I'm saying that in order to feel, that we must be saying words, either out loud or in our head, then how can I also be saying feelings happen to us only when we are beyond words?

The answer begins with taking what I've just said literally. To wit, the first three truths require we *describe something with words*. With facts, our words describe what we've physically measured. With stories, they describe experiences wherein these measurements occurred. And with ideas, they describe the abstract essence of these measurement stories. With feelings, though, the words we say *are what we are describing*. Do you get the difference? Like all things about feelings, seeing this can be tough at first.

Essentially the difference lies in how we arrive at these words. With facts, stories, and ideas, we arrive at the words *by* measuring, narrating, or theorizing. But with feelings, we arrive at the words *by being unable to* measure, narrate, or theorize. In other words, we arrive at them only after those kinds of words fail.

This failure then creates the spiritual hole I've been referring to. And if we stay in this experience, all manner of non logical emanations begin to emerge, including the sounds of words used as feelings.

Here, a good example would be the word *om*. The American Heritage® Dictionary of the English Language, Fourth Edition, describes this well known Hindu word as *The supreme and most sacred syllable in Hinduism & Buddhism, consisting in Sanskrit of the three sounds (a), (u), and (m), representing various fundamental triads and believed to be the spoken essence of the universe. It is uttered as a mantra and in affirmations and blessings.*

Once again, we're referring to something believed to describe the entire nature of the universe. Deep definition, eh? Those who favor the spiritual wise man are probably enjoying all this. The main thing to see however is how differently the word *om* is used from normal words. In effect, when Hindus and Buddhists chant *om*, this word has a dual nature. First, this word carries them beyond ordinary words. Second, this word expresses what they feel when they arrive at this state beyond words— when they're feeling the spiritual essence of life; when they reach their feelings.

For Hindus and Buddhists then, the word *om* both creates the space for feelings and becomes the way the mind and body voice these feelings. Hence my saying the word *om* has a dual nature. Moreover, to be considered feelings, we must be using words in this special way. On the one hand, our words must carry us past our normal sense of words. And on the other, they must express what we're feeling when we are finally past those words.

How Similar Feelings Blend Together Over Time

Now we're going to address something which confuses a lot of people—the idea that we literally cannot tell when our feelings begin or end. Sometimes this problem is merely laughable, such as when we feel we'll love someone forever and all that wonderful craziness. But when our feelings are painful, such as when someone insults us or worse, this can lead us to overestimate people's malevolence and then, to grossly overreact.

Where do these overreactions come from? In part they come from our tendency to store and compartmentalize unresolved feelings, good and bad alike. We'll talk a lot about this in Book II when we address the nature of resentment. The real problem however is not resentment per se. Rather it's that we cannot place our feelings in the field of time, other than to vaguely reference a logically approximate time.

The thing to notice here is the way we use the word "time." In these instances, we're not referring to time itself. Rather, we're referring to "events," such as the time such and such happened. Not getting this? Then think back to the last "time" you felt angry. Now ask yourself, was all of your anger coming from what happened to you then? Or did it include feelings from other times as well?

Because we have no way to know when our feelings begin or end, most people assume the former. Yet we frequently see examples wherein people act irrationally—or make big deals out of seemingly insignificant events—all because what they're currently feeling reminds them of things they felt in previous events, feelings that occurred in other "times."

In Book III, we'll discuss how to find and resolve these kinds of feelings. You'll be surprised by how easy it is to do. For now, however, the thing to ask is, can we even know if what we're currently feeling is connected to what's happening in the present? Oddly, a lot of unnecessary pain and confusion—as well as a lot of truly bad therapy—stems from not focusing more on this question.

The answer to this question is also easy to find. But to arrive at this answer, we need to use an idea most scientists consider nonsense. We need to use psychophysics.

Using Psychophysics to Help Us Understand Feelings

What is psychophysics? It's the belief that all things in our world, both material and immaterial, are governed by the same basic set of laws.

Today's scientists see this belief as crazy. Yet no less than Einstein, Niels Bohr, Sigmund Freud, William James, Carl Jung, and a slew of other geniuses whose work is still considered brilliant openly acknowledged their belief in psychophysics. Why raise this controversy in the section on feelings? Because even folks who have never heard of this idea tend to use it, every time they equate the properties of their feelings—and the properties of most things they call spiritual—with the natural properties of analogous physical world objects.

For instance, take the idea of trying to understand the nature of feelings. For thousands of years, spiritual teachers have equated the properties of feelings with the properties of water, from Chinese philosophers (one of the five elements) and Persian astrologers (water signs) to the great African poet, Birago Diop, who so beautifully described the feelings we have about those who have died: *Those who are dead never left. They are in the trickling of water. They are sleeping in water. The dead are not dead. Hear more often, the murmur of things, not people. Hear the voice of water.*

So can we use psychophysics to better understand the nature of our feelings? Absolutely. And to do this, just imagine there is a bowl of clear water in front of you, and an eye dropper filled with red ink lying next to it. Now imagine you will be squeezing one droplet of this red ink into this bowl each time you feel angry. Can you picture doing this? Droplets of red ink will be going into a bowl of clear water.

Now imagine you're out to dinner and someone pisses you off. Perhaps the maître d' calls you stupid. In goes one drop of red ink. Now imagine a second person does something to make you mad. Perhaps your wife calls you stupid for getting so mad at the maître d' for calling you stupid. In goes a second drop of red ink. Finally, imagine a third person does something. Maybe in the midst of criticizing your response to the maître d', your waiter knocks spaghetti and meat balls onto your new Dior Homme suit. Only one more drop of ink, you think? It feels like it deserves a whole freakin' bowl full of red ink. But rules are rules. So in goes one drop.

Now imagine it's several days later and you are sitting with your therapist. You have just told her the story of these three insults, and she has asked you how you feel about the waiter ruining your new suit. Would you be able to answer? In other words, could you feel your spaghetti-on-the-suit anger without feeling the other two angers as well?

The answer is in the bowl of water. Just as we cannot separate drops of red ink once they go into a bowl of water, we cannot separate similar feelings from separate events either. Hence our tendency to over or underreact and when we do, to justify our feelings with reasons. We feel similar feelings cumulatively.

Do Dissimilar Feelings Blend Together as Well?

What I've just said is that we can't separate similar feelings which occur in different events. So is this true for dissimilar feelings as well? Do feelings always blend together? Here again, psychophysics holds the answer.

This time imagine you are looking at sunlight passing though a prism. Now imagine trying to see the entire scene and at the same time, only the red colored rays. Can you do it? If you've never tried this, the answer may surprise you. You won't be able to do it. You will of course be able to picture the whole prism as one object. And if you really try, you'll be able to focus on just the red colored rays. But you won't be able to focus on both at the same time, at least not for long, and certainly not without going blank.

Why can't we do this? It turns out that the more we focus on one color, the less we see the rest. And the more we try to take in all the colors, the less we can see the individual colors. Moreover, this inability—to see the parts and the whole simultaneously—is not a flaw in us. Rather it's part of how we experience everything in the real world, including our feelings.

Are you having trouble getting what I'm saying? Then try this. Imagine it's night and that you are in a large wedding hall with many lights, all turned on. Now imagine one of these many lights is red, and the rest are the usual white. So let me ask you. What determines how much red light you'll see? The answer, of course, is where you focus. The more you focus on the one red light, the less white light you'll see. But if you look away from this one red light, you'll barely see any red light at all.

What keeps us from seeing the red light? In a word, diffusion, something which happens to many similar classes of real world things. And not to dissimilar ones. Said in lay terms, similar classes of real world things tend to blend together when put in the same container—water soluble dyes and colored light being two common examples. Indeed, this is what prevents us from seeing the red light when we try to take in the whole room. It diffuses into the total light in the room. Similarly, the drops of red ink which diffuse into the bowl of clear water, and the red colored rays of the prism which diffuse into the whole picture in our mind.

The point is, diffusion also affects the way we sense feelings, which is why it takes so much effort to feel only certain feelings. If we narrow our focus, we can do this, just as we can focus on the red light. But if we don't, we experience our whole spiritual self, similar to the way we see the whole prism, and the whole bowl of water, and the whole lit room.

Can we consciously experience two or more feelings at a time then? Yes, but not as separate feelings. And to see this, we'll need to do yet another psychophysical thought experiment, this time with a brand new box of Crayola's. We'll use the childhood dream-box size, 128 crayons. Here, our feelings will be represented by the various colored crayons which, if you remember, arrive sorted by color, similar colors together.

So now, let me ask you. How hard is it to look at two dissimilar crayons and simultaneously see them both clearly? Do you find that your eyes tend to flip back and forth? Annoying, isn't it? The point is, we can either see the whole box of crayons or each crayon separately. But we can't see both. And we can't see dissimilar crayons separately at the same time.

This then answers our question as to whether we can feel two or more dissimilar feelings at a time. The answer is, to a limited degree, we can, but not without the annoying property of switching back and forth.

We can also note the intensity of our overall emotional state and zoom in on one specific feeling—for instance—on our feelings of anger. But since feelings diffuse, we cannot do both. Nor can we feel two separate feelings, both at the same time.

What Determines the Amount of Pain We Feel?

Speaking of focusing on individual feelings, let me ask you something. Did you know that suffering acknowledged—the suffering we focus on—is the source of most feelings? And that unacknowledged suffering—the suffering we do not focus on—is more an idea than anything else?

This explains why focusing away from suffering decreases pain. To begin with, the word *pain* is just another way to refer to suffering acknowledged—the suffering we focus on. And unacknowledged suffering is pain changed into ideas.

So why does unacknowledged pain hurt less? Because ideas are an off-switch for feelings. Thus, by converting painful feelings into ideas about painful feelings, we turn off some of these painful feelings.

A good thing to keep in mind about pain then is that, the more we focus on it, the more we feel it—and the less we focus on it, the less we feel it. This is but one of the implications of the diagram on page 83, *The Master Continuum of Feelings*. Or to state this in the language of the rationalist wise man, the perceived size of our pain is directly proportionate to the overall dynamic range of our current spiritual life. Spiritual life is the rationalist wise man's way to refer to feelings, remember?

This means, the broader the overall range of our spiritual life, the more diffused our feelings will be, and the less we will suffer. Whereas the narrower the range, the deeper our feelings will be, and the more we'll suffer.

This explains why alcoholics—and extremely depressed people—can cry profusely and yet feel almost no pain. Their spiritual life is so diffused that people witnessing them often feel more pain than they do. It also explains how we can work on our spiritual condition for years, and at times, hurt worse. Unless, of course, we use the off-switch quality of facts, stories, and ideas to manage our feelings.

To Learn About Feelings, Try Meditating on Holes

Speaking of ways to better manage your spiritual life, a good part of doing this requires you keep in mind how spiritual words serve dual duty. In effect, spiritual words serve two roles. They creates holes and they express what comes out of these holes. Sounds complicated, right? The thing is, we already use quite a few of these words, albeit, not in ways which get us in touch with our feelings. Chaos. Infinity. God. The abyss. The Ineffable. The hole. The Oneness. Used correctly, all these words can get us in touch with our feelings.

Of course, for this to happen, you must first know how to use these words to create the space for feelings. For instance, take the word *hole*. For thousands of years, societies have been using this image to represent the spiritual origin of all things. Yet if you wanted to define the spiritual nature of the word *hole*, what would you say? That holes are where our feelings emerge from, and that what is around these holes—our ideas, facts, and stories—are the rest?

Okay. This is true. Precise, even. But there's a problem. This description is an idea. Thus it can't teach us much about accessing our feelings.

Is there a way to get past this problem then?

Here again, psychophysics comes to our rescue, by giving us a foothold into this admittedly deep concept. To wit, if you meditate on the physical properties of holes—first, by envisioning something physical with a hole in it, then, by gradually removing what is around this hole until all you have left is the hole—what you'll be left with is your feelings. And this makes sense, yes? Holes are where our feelings come from. So the better you get at sensing holes, the more access you'll have to your feelings.

Why does this happen? Because meditating on removing what surrounds a hole functions like a Zen koan—a story, dialogue, question, or statement, the meaning of which can't be understood by rational thinking, but which may be accessible through intuition. Thus like all koans, meditating on holes will cause you to exceed the limits of your ability to put something into words. By doing this, you'll access the source of your feelings. Indeed, the more you attempt to remove what you can see around holes, the more feelings you will feel. An interesting way to get in touch with your spiritual self, to be sure. As well as a wonderful introduction to Zen practice.

One More John Story—How Laughter Kills Pain

Finally, speaking of learning ways to better manage your feelings, and as a fitting closing to this chapter, I want to tell you another John story. In this story, one feeling—laughter—displaced another—severe physical pain. At the time, John had suffered extreme burns over a good portion of his body and had just been admitted to a hospital. So bad were his burns that the flesh on his arms was falling off. Can you imagine the pain? I cannot.

At one point, during the admission, a male nurse, a man John had known from high school, had to perform some rather intimate procedures on him. At which point, John quipped, "I guess this means we'll have to get married."

My point for telling you this? I've regressed John to this scene several times and he always laughs out loud. Moreover, try as he may, he cannot feel pain in this moment. Nor, John states, did he feel any at this point in the original event. Thus in the midst of what had to have been the worst pain of his life, laughter displaced anguish. More proof for that we can feel only one feeling at a time—and more evidence that the spiritual wise man has his merits, one of them being that laughter is one of life's most powerful forces.

Comedy as a Feeling

As you probably realize by now—and as the spiritual wise man is fond of pointing out—comedy is a class of feelings. Moreover, with these feelings, he somehow manages to temporarily subjugate the other three wise men into being delivery boys for his truth, as in fact-based comedy, story-based comedy, and idea-based comedy. This is why I'll be offering no examples this time, as all comedy is spiritual comedy. Then again, anyone who has had a good laugh in the midst of feeling severe physical or psychological pain knows just how powerful spiritual comedy can be. As I mentioned a moment ago, the pain goes away. At least while you're laughing.

How powerful is that?

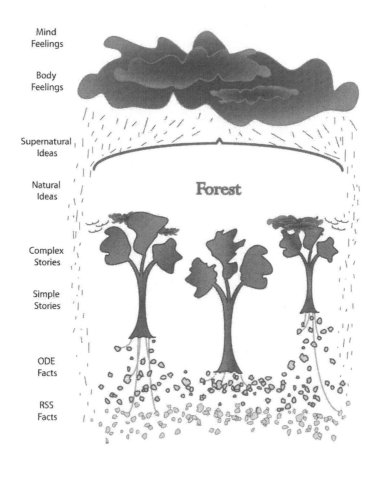

The Life Cycle of
the Four Great Truths

Mind
Feelings

Body
Feelings

Supernatural
Ideas

Natural
Ideas

Forest

Complex
Stories

Simple
Stories

ODE
Facts

RSS
Facts

The Forest Metaphor—a Good Way to Remember All This

Is your head ready to burst open from the amount of information I've just bombarded you with? I know. In a book on too-much-information, this can seem insensitive. And downright dumb. The good news is, everything in this chapter can be summarized in a single drawing. And if you look at the drawing on the opposite page, what you'll find is just such a drawing.

The thing to keep in mind, of course, is how picturing is the key to finding personal truth. Including that this psychophysical story is yet one more example of how ideas come alive when you picture them. Here, the life cycle of a forest—and how it comes into being—is seen as a parallel to how the four great truths come into being. How so?

Facts are like *soil*. Thus RSSs (references to a standard scale) are like the nutrients in the soil. ODEs (observations of definite events) are then like decaying real world matter which combines with these nutrients to make fertile soil.

Stories are like *trees*. Stories grow in this soil. Thus all stories are like trees rooted in facts. A simple story is like a tree with three main branches of roots (three related ODEs). A complex story adds to this birds (ideas), clouds (feelings), and more roots (extra facts).

Ideas are like our *view* from above the forest. Here the word *view* is the key. Natural ideas are like the words we might use to describe this view to a friend, and supernatural ideas are like the technical language we might use to explain what we see to a scientist.

Finally, feelings are like the *rain clouds* which keep the forest lush. Here, body feelings are like the clouds themselves, and mind feelings are like the rain which gets absorbed into the soil and activates the nutrients.

Overall, the thing to notice here is how something which occurs in the real world—a forest—can so mirror the relationships between what we experience everyday and what I've been calling the four great truths. No surprise then that these relationships underlie everything in our world, including human personality. Thus the more you learn to see these relationships, the more connected you'll feel to everything around you. And the more connected you become, the more you'll have the life you want. The life you so deserve.

All you need do is remember the forest.

Notes Written in the Margins of Chapter Two

My Use of the Word *God*

Some folks may notice I've chosen to use the word *God* several times in this chapter. Know this mirrors the way I speak in life. At the same time, at the risk of offending many, like Joseph Campbell, I openly admit to not believing in a personal god, a god who is so small as to be fashioned in a human being's likeness and image, only with superpowers.

I mention this as I do not want people to think I am biased toward a religious perspective, nor toward the spiritual wise man. Rather, while I love learning about people's religions, and about spiritual things in general, I myself see whatever created us as being similar to everything else I've described in the feelings section—ineffable, unknowable, and beyond words.

At the same time, I frequently voice this ineffable, unknowable, indescribable force in terms which I hope will make my ideas better understood. These terms frequently include words from other people's philosophies and religious beliefs. That I voice my ideas this way does not imply I endorse anyone else's truth. It means only that I admire, honor, and respect other people's beliefs, especially the parts of their philosophical, religious, and spiritual beliefs which teach us to love each other more.

Why *Three* Core Qualities of Truth?

One of the things I've used to define the four great truths is something I call the *three core qualities*. To be honest, I know this title sounds a bit grand. Where do these three core qualities come from anyway? And why three, and not four or seventy one? The answer is simple. Like all things in our world, all truths—both physical or non physical alike—are psychophysical. They are governed by the same set of laws. Thus, because our physical truths are based on these three core qualities, our non physical truths must be as well.

What are the three core qualities of physical truths? Time, place, and change. Or stated a bit more formally, reference time, the inertial frame of reference (time in relationship to space), plus any observed movement.

Obviously, there are a lot of things we could propose, state, and argue as to how these three qualities do or do not define our physical world. My only point for raising this though is that these same three core qualities are the three core psychophysical elements present in all truths, physical and non physical alike. Hence my choice to use these three core qualities—a reference time frame, a reference place frame, and a reference experience—to define the four great truths.

Afterthoughts on My Decision to Define the Four Great Truths

Facts. Feelings. Stories. Ideas. When I began this chapter, my goal seemed simple—define each of these four great truths. When I found myself struggling to find the words to do this though, I realized how naive I had been. In effect, I'd agreed to divide all we say, think, feel, and do—all of being itself—into just four piles. In one chapter, no less. But just as this chapter was beginning to feel like I was writing war and peace, I remembered a word. Ontology.

What is *ontology*? In case you've managed to avoid having to take philosophy 101, ontology means the study of *being* itself. So what does "being" mean? God knows. Folks a lot smarter than I have been trying to put this idea into words for millennia now.

Why mention this? Because I once again want to make sure you give yourself credit for getting through this chapter, regardless of how many times your mind went blank. Ontological discussions entail some of the most difficult ideas in all of human history. Anyone doubting this should try reading Wittgenstein's *Tractatus Logico-Philosophicus*.

My point is, given half a brain, I probably should have looked harder for a way around this chapter. Reading it has to have been tough. Writing it certainly was. Unfortunately for both of us, there is no way around this chapter. All truth rests on these four concepts. And while agreeing to define *being* itself is probably not one of my better ideas, the difference between insanity and genius is slim at times. Hopefully this will ultimately turn out to be a time wherein this slim margin ends up in my favor.

Resources for Chapter Two—Meet the Four Wise Men

Abraham Lincoln (1809-1865)

Wills, Gary. (1992). *Lincoln at Gettysburg, The Words That Remade America*. New York: Touchstone / Simon & Schuster. (In the section on ideas, I referred to Lincoln's "I don't need a law" speech. You'll find this speech on pages 93-95. To be honest, when I first read it, I was upset by what I read. In time though, I came to regard this as a good example of Lincoln's absolute gift for tact—in this case, sending racists to hell while having them smile on their way. A terrific book and one that certainly deserved the Pulitzer Prize it garnered.)

Spiritual Wisdoms

Borg, Marcus. (2006). *Jesus, Uncovering the Life, Teachings, and Relevance of a Religious Revolutionary*. San Francisco: Harper Collins. (I find this one of the best books for exploring how the Jesus of history and the Jesus of faith differ. Borg is respectful, insightful, and thought provoking.)

Barratt, George J. (2008). *The Origin of the Yin Yang Symbol*. London: Lulu Press. (For anyone interested in the science behind this symbol, this is a clear, short e-book which patiently explains the shadow acquisition process from which the Tao symbol is derived.)

Capra, Fritjof. (1999). *The Tao of Physics, An Exploration of the Parallels Between Modern Physics and Eastern Mysticism, 25th Anniversary Edition*. Boston: Shambhala. (I consider Capra to be one of the clearest thinkers ever. Descartes would certainly approve of his writings. What I mentioned about Niels Bohr's family crest came from this book.)

Dale, Ralph Alan. (2004, 2002). *Tao Te Ching, A New Translation & Commentary*. New York: Barnes & Noble. Watkins Publishing. (For those interested, a visually beautiful edition with a thoughtful translation and a wonderful preface.)

Ludwig Wittgenstein (1889-1951)

Wittgenstein, Ludwig. (1922, 2003). *Tractatus Logico-Philosophicus*. Library of Essential Reading Series. C. K. Ogden (Trans.), Bertrand Russell (Introduction). New York: Barnes and Noble. (If you insist, this is a good translation.)

Strathern, Paul. (1996). *Wittgenstein in 90 Minutes*. Chicago: Ivan R. Dee. (Anything by Paul Strathern is pithy and gets into the cracks and under the cupboard. As readable an introduction to Wittgenstein as you can find. Or better yet, listen to the Blackstone Audio version, 2003.)

Odds & Ends

Bo Derek co-starred with Dudley Moore in Blake Edwards 1979 film 10, for which she received a Golden Globe nomination for best actress.

Paul Newman won an Academy award for his 1967 performance in Cool Hand Luke.

Diop, Birago. (1967). *Leurres et lueurs, poèmes, 2nd ed*. Paris: Présence Africaine. (The Diop poem I've quoted has several translations. The one I've used I gleaned from the net and believe this book to be the original source.)

"'With An Even Hand,' Brown V. Board of Education at Fifty." (2004). Washington, DC: Library of Congress. <http://www.loc.gov/exhibits/brown> (A good description of how folks with the courage to speak their personal truth can provoke social change.)

Fleck, Ludwick. (1979, 1935). *Genesis and Development of a Scientific Fact*. Chicago: University of Chicago Press.

Chapter 3

Arranging Words—The Wise Men's Map

A First Look at the Map of the Mind

Having introduced you to the four wise men, I now need to tell you about where they live—the four realms of truth. Here, I'm referring to the Material Realm, the Empirical Realm, the Rational Realm, and the Spiritual Realm. And lest it's not clear where these four realms are, they exist in the map of the mind I referred to in chapter one.

Know that the metaphysical boundaries which divide these four realms much resemble the physical geography which defines most countries. In both cases, the boundaries derive mainly from naturally occurring features. In the physical world, we're talking about things like rivers, deserts, forests, and mountains. But in the world of the four wise men, there are only two natural features—a horizontal boundary called the Real World to Theoretical World Axis, and a vertical boundary called the Mind Body Axis.

In addition, at the intersection of these two boundaries, there's a sort of neutral meeting ground called the Axis Mundi. Here you'll find The Hall of Wisdom, the one place in the whole world wherein you can find your personal truth. And yes, you can find pieces of your truth in all four of the wise men's realms. But only in The Hall of Wisdom can you make this truth your own.

Of course, to locate the The Hall of Wisdom, you must understand the map. This begins with learning about the four realms of truth. The goal of this chapter then will be to teach you the lay of the land in and around the Axis Mundi, beginning with an overview.

Please keep in mind that reaching the Axis Mundi is just the beginning of finding your personal truth. You will still have to learn how to sit with the four wise men without being taken in or losing yourself. For now though, we're going to focus only on gaining an overall sense of the four realms, beginning with the map on the opposite page.

The Four Realms of Truth

Does this map look familiar? It should. It very much resembles the northern European, pre-Christian symbol I mentioned in the last chapter—the Celtic cross. In both cases, the entire world exists within a circle divided by two perpendicular lines, the end-points of which refer to the four directions.

With the map of the four realms, of course, these two lines also define the boundaries of the four wise men's territories. Moreover, along with the Axis Mundi, each adjacent pair of end-points defines the nature of a realm. For instance, take the southeast realm. Here you'll find the first of the four great truths—facts. And to see the nature of this truth, you combine the Axis Mundi with the two adjacent end-points. Thus facts are theoretical truths about physical things, including the body.

Now let's do this for the northwest realm. Here we find the fourth of the four great truths—feelings. And the nature of this truth? Combining the Axis Mundi with the two end-points, we see that feelings are real world truths about non physical things, including the mind.

Moving now to the southwest realm, we find the second of the four great truths—stories. And if we consult the map, we find that stories are real world truths about physical things, including the body.

Finally, in the northeast realm, we find the third of the four great truths—ideas. And according to the map, ideas are theoretical truths about non physical things, including the mind.

Now let's take a closer look at the two boundary lines which define these four truths, beginning with the horizontal boundary line, the Real World to Theoretical World Axis.

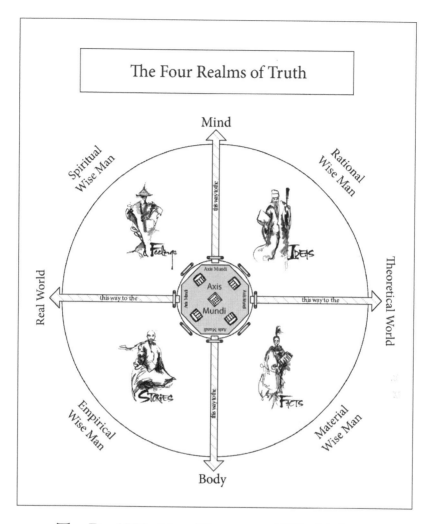

The Real World to Theoretical World Axis
(the horizontal boundary)

Descartes tells us we can either be certain of a truth or we can be certain we cannot know it. And when you understand the nature of the horizontal axis, you know why he is right. Oddly, most people today embrace only one of these two viewpoints. Either they believe in *real world truth*, meaning we can at best increment toward an ultimately unreachable truth. Or they believe in *theoretical truth*, meaning, if we keep trying, we can come to know all of a certain truth.

In effect, those who believe in real world truth believe the whole truth can never be known. However, by continuing to move toward this whole truth, we can learn to better manage our lives. Whereas those who believe in theoretical truth believe that beneath everything, there are knowable laws and principles—moreover, that if we look long enough, we can come to know the entire nature of this truth.

In reality, both groups are right, which is why personal truths must include both of Descartes' viewpoints. And to see why, we're once again going to turn to psychophysics, this time using the nature of coins to reveal the five ways in which the horizontal axis defines personal truth.

How the Horizontal Axis Defines Personal Truth

How does the nature of the horizontal axis resemble that of coins? Just as one sided coins cannot exist, neither can one sided truths. Thus, like coins, truth must have two opposite sides. At the same time, because we can never know the nature of a coin from seeing only one side, to know the nature of a coin, we must treat these two sides as a single entity. Personal truths require we do this as well.

Here then are the first two ways in which the horizontal axis defines personal truth. First, all personal truths must juxtapose two opposite viewpoints. Moreover the nature of this juxtaposition is that one truth must be a theoretical truth (the whole truth is knowable) while the other must be a real world truth (the whole truth is not knowable). Second, to arrive at a personal truth, we must treat these two viewpoints as one continuum of truth. Here, these two viewpoints, and all those inbetween, are simultaneously possible and true.

This then leads us to the third way in which the horizontal axis defines personal truth. While the mind can easily grasp the idea that one coin has two sides (a theoretical truth), we can never see both sides of a coin simultaneously (a real world truth). The same idea holds true for personal truth as well. While in theory, we can know a whole personal truth, in the real world, there will always be one side we cannot see.

Here again, we find evidence that Descartes was right. We can either be certain of a truth, or we can be certain we cannot know it. Said as a function of the horizontal axis, this means that while we can know that both kinds of truths exist, we can never see both truths at the same time. One will always remain unknowable—the side we cannot see.

Some would now ask why we can't accumulate what we see in successive turns of the coin. And in theory, we can. But in the real world, summing what we see on two sides of a coin is never the same as seeing both sides simultaneously. Here again, we'll need to turn to psychophysics to see why.

Picture a cake. Now ask yourself this. Can you taste each ingredient separately, then sum the results to know how this cake will taste? Or say you are doing an oil painting of flowers in a vase. Can you paint each flower separately, then sum the results to complete the painting?

In theory, we should be able to do both these things. In theory, the sum of the parts equals the whole. But in the real world, the whole is always more than the sum of the parts. Thus the fourth way in which the horizontal axis defines personal truth lies in knowing how sums add up. Theoretical sums add up to the whole. Real world sums do not.

And the fifth aspect? It's the technical explanation for why we cannot know the entire nature of anything by summing the parts. You see, unlike the theoretical nature of a thing—which we can get from summing the parts—the real world nature of a thing is always an emergent quality. In other words, while the theoretical nature of a thing can be deduced from logic, experimentation, and reasoning, the real world nature of this thing emerges only when we take it in as a whole.

Not sure of what I'm saying? Let's turn to psychophysics once more.

Consider the nature of water. Good old H_2O. If we separate water into its two base elements—hydrogen and oxygen—both are combustible. But taken as a whole, water is not only noncombustible. It puts out fires.

My point is, the noncombustible quality of water emerges only when we observe it as a whole. Moreover, we could never predict that water would be like this by observing the nature of the parts separately. If we could, logically, water should burn. But it doesn't.

That it doesn't is called an emergent property—a property present only in the whole.

Which Truth Is Better, Theoretical or Real World?

In a moment, I'll summarize these five aspects of the horizontal axis. Before I do, let me ask you. Are you beginning to see, how, in order to arrive at a personal truth, we must juxtapose a theoretical truth with a real world truth? More important, can you see why we also need the continuum in between?

So which end of this continuum more resembles the way you look for truth? The theoretical world end wherein, if you look long and hard enough, you can discover the truth about pretty much anything? If so, know you're in good company. Indeed, were you to study the lives of the greatest minds, you'd find a long list of folks who would agree with you. Parmenides and Kant. Descartes and Newton. Plank and Einstein. Chomsky and Darwin.

At the same time, you would also find great minds who, although considered by some to be theorists, advocated more for the real world end of this continuum. Heraclitus and Hume. Bacon and da Vinci. Heisenberg and Bohr. Capra and Hawking.

Even here though, to truly understand who these folks are, you must juxtapose theoretical to real world opposites. For instance, take Francis Bacon, considered by many to be the catalyst for the scientific revolution. In his *Novum Organum* (New Instrument), published in 1620, he argues that inductive reasoning—generalizing from real world observations to axioms to laws—is the only way to arrive at truth. And in the real world, he is right. At the same time, Descartes argued that we cannot trust our senses, that our senses lie, and that to find a truth we must eliminate any and all doubt. And in theory, he is right too.

Obviously, then, both men are right—Descartes in theory, and Bacon in the real world. Yet according to Bacon, Descartes could not be right. He had no real world proof. And according to Descartes, this lack of real world proof was irrelevant. And indeed Descartes was right as well.

Here then is a good example of how theoretical truths and real world truths can conflict. Moreover, when you understand the horizontal axis, you understand how Descartes' idea—that truth is either clear and distinct or unknowable, so clearly represents this conflict. You also understand how so many folks can argue that genuine truth should be the same in all places and times, when in reality, no such universal truth exists. At least none we humans can personally witness. Moreover, to find your personal truth, you'll need to learn to see the good in both these truths.

In Book III, we'll return to these ideas and explore them in depth, when we talk about how the combination of two principles of modern physics—Werner Heisenberg's uncertainty principle, and Niels Bohr's complementarity principle, lead to this same conclusion. In addition, we'll also look at how you can combine these two principles to form a clear and distinct test for personal truth. And yes, grasping the full implications of these two principles can be a bit tough at first. After all, both men are bonafide geniuses. However, once you see how naturally these two ideas fit together, I'm sure you'll do just fine.

By the way, if you're feeling a bit overwhelmed by all this intellectual stuff, allow me to remind you of what the famous American baseball player, manager, and dugout philosopher, Yogi Berra, once said. *In theory, there is no difference between theory and practice. But in practice, there is.*

A pretty good synopsis of the Real World to Theoretical World axis, if I do say so myself. Go, Yogi.

Summarizing the Horizontal Axis

Now let's summarize what I've just told you about the horizontal axis, starting with that there are five ways in which the Real World to Theoretical World Axis defines personal truth.

Duality
There are two kinds of truth on the horizontal axis, theoretical and real world.

First, the horizontal axis represents the most basic quality in our world—duality. All coins have two sides. All truths do as well. Moreover, with personal truth, the two sides of this duality come from juxtaposing a theoretical truth with a real world truth.

Unity
Together, these two kinds of truth comprise the horizontal axis.

theoretical truth   real world truth

Second, the horizontal axis also represents the experience of unity, the theoretical truth from which all dualities emerge. Thus while all coins have two sides, all coins are also single objects. As are all truths. With personal truth, we take the two truths we've juxtaposed in step one and use them as the end points of a single continuum. Here, a pair of opposites creates a unity of possible truths. This continuum extends from the complete predictability of theoretical truths on one end all the way to the complete unpredictability of real world truths on the other.

Simultaneity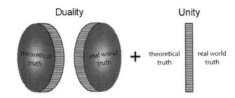
To find a personal
truth, we must
remain aware of
both aspects
simultaneously.

Third, the horizontal axis tells us that to know a personal truth, we must be simultaneously aware of all three viewpoints—the two dualities (the two sides) and the unity (the one coin). In theory, we can do this. In the real world, we cannot.

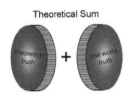

Sums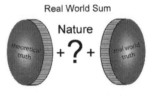
In theory, the whole
equals the sum of
the parts. In the real
world, the whole
equals more.

The fourth aspect of the horizontal line then explains why we can do this only in theory. It states, while in theory, the whole equals the sum of the parts, in the real world, the whole is always more than this sum.

Emergent Properties
Some parts of the
horizontal axis are
visible only when a
thing is in its
natural state.

This then leads us to the idea which explains why the fourth aspect exists—the existence of emergent properties. In this, the fifth aspect of the horizontal axis, we see that there are properties which exist only when a thing is in its whole, natural state—moreover, that when a thing is in its theoretical state, these emergent properties disappear.

Using the Five Aspects to Define Personal Truth

In a moment, we're going to look at how these five aspects also define the vertical axis. Before we do, I need to restate them once more. Only this time, I'm going to voice them as general statements about personal truth. Can you guess what they are? It's simpler than you might imagine.

[1] Duality—All personal truth is grounded in duality. All coins have two sides.

[2] Unity—All duality stems from a unity. All personal truths do as well. Thus while all coins do indeed have two sides, all coins are simultaneously a single object.

[3] Simultaneity—To arrive at personal truth, we must keep in mind both the unity and the duality. All coins are simultaneously one coin with two sides.

[4] Sums—In theory, we can do this, by summing the unity with the duality. In the real world, we cannot. Thus personal truths are always more than the sum of the prior three aspects. Here, theoretical sums are one truth, real world sums the other, and both together make a third truth. But what you see on the two sides of a coin can't be summed to a whole truth.

[5] Emergent Properties—The idea of emergent properties explains why we can't sum these three truths to find personal truth. The nature of real world things exists only when they are in their natural state. *This makes personal truth an emergent quality, the result of the simultaneously experienced combination of theoretical world truth plus real world truth.* Hence the difference between a real world truth and a theoretical truth.

Now let's look at how these five aspects define the vertical axis—the Mind Body Axis. What is a *mind* anyway, and what is a *body*? Obviously there has been a lot of nonsense spewed as to what these two things are, including the materialist wise man's belief that the mind does not exist. If we set these objections aside though and look at how the five aspects of personal truth apply to the Mind Body Axis, we begin to see what makes people fall for this kind of sanctimonious twaddle. We also get to see what has made it so hard for us to understand things like addictions and learning disabilities.

The Mysterious Mind Body Axis (the vertical boundary)

Toward the end of the previous chapter, I briefly mentioned that to understand the nature of personal truth, we must understand mind body dualism—moreover, that to understand mind body dualism, we must

The Five Aspects
as Qualities of Personal Truth

Duality
All coins have two sides.

Duality
All personal truth is
grounded in duality.

Unity
These two sides make one
coin. Thus while all coins do
indeed have two sides, all
coins are simultaneously a
single object.

Unity
All duality stems from a
unity. All personal truths
do as well.

Simultaneity
All coins are simultaneously
one coin with two sides.

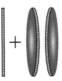

Simultaneity
To arrive at personal truth, we
must keep in mind both the
unity and the duality.

Sums
What you see on the two
sides of a coin can't be
summed to a whole.

Sums
In theory, we can sum the prior
three truths. In the real world, we
cannot. Thus personal truths are
always more than the sum of the
prior three aspects.

Emergent Properties
The real world nature of a
coin emerges only when
it is whole.

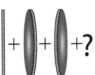

Emergent Properties
The idea of emergent properties
explains why we can't sum these
three truths to find personal truth.
The real world nature of things
exists only when they exist in their
natural state.

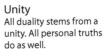

remember that the mind processes information more quickly than the body. Heady as all this seems, it all boils down to one thing.

The speed at which we process our sensations determines where in ourselves we look for truth. Here, the faster we process life, the more we seek truth in the mind—and the slower we process life, the more we seek truth in the body.

In the next chapter, we'll look at the biological and psychological evidence for how these time-based differences affect our ability to find truth. Why go through all this trouble? Because the answers to many mysteries lie in understanding how the mind and body process life at different speeds.

For instance, take compulsions and addictions. What is the one thing all addictions and compulsions have in common? They rapidly and predictably alter the speed at which you sense time. Moreover, this experience is what you get addicted to—to the experience of being able to speed time up or slow it down. This is why we call them uppers and downers, remember?

This explains how we can sometimes get hooked on people, places, things, and events. We get hooked on these things because being around them significantly alters our sense of time. Moreover, because the Mind Body Axis is the source of your sense of personal time, to understand why these things happen, you'll need to understand the Mind Body Axis.

Another mystery the Mind Body Axis explains is why some folks are naturally good at sports, dance, and music, while others of us downright suck at body-based learning activities. Again, if you understand how the speed at which you process life affects physical activities differently from mental ones, you know why. Briefly stated, because the mind by nature processes life more quickly than the body, when your mind races ahead, your body can't keep up. For example, have you ever tried to give someone directions while simultaneously trying to draw a map? It doesn't work too well, does it. How about trying to learn a new dance step by mentally telling your feet where to go? How many left feet do you have? And how about thinking your way through a video game rather than just letting your body react? Did you say your two year old can beat you?

Not surprisingly, Yogi Berra had something profound to say about this too—that *you can't think and bat*. And indeed, here again, Yogi is right. You can't think and bat. Why not? Because the mind processes time more quickly than the body, the result of the laws of physics. Thus when you're doing a physical activity and hear your mind telling you how to do it, in effect, you're hearing instructions from two different bosses, one boss who is telling you, "hurry up and get it done," and a second boss who is telling you, "take your time and do it right." Ever try to follow instructions from two bosses at once and do anything well? Again, to grasp what's happening here, you'll need to understand the Mind Body Axis.

Of course, like all truths, to understand this one, you'll need to look at the complementary truth as well. Here, the complementary truth might go something like, *you can't bat and think.* What the heck does this mean? Well think about it. What is the opposite of body-based learning activities? Mind-based learning activities. And what do we say about folks who physically struggle in mind-based learning settings? That they have ADHD.

What does the Mind Body Axis have to do with having ADHD? Well, would you believe, a good portion of the problems folks with ADHD encounter in classrooms stem from a mismatch between the rate at which they hear ideas and the rate at which teachers speak? Simply put, people whose normal processing speed exists at the body end of the Mind Body Axis need to be spoken to more slowly, as these folks tend to process words in their body first and only later, in their mind.

If this is you, then your body will tend to hear things before your mind understands them. Moreover, because body-based processes take more time than mind-based processes—and because the bias in education leans toward teaching more and faster—if you're given more time to process words, you'll likely learn a lot more.

In later chapters, we'll be exploring these mysteries in depth. For any of this to make sense to you though, you'll first need to understand the vertical axis. This means we'll need to look at how the five aspects of personal truth—Duality, Unity, Simultaneity, Sums, and Emergent Properties—apply to that axis. And while this may get a bit hairy, referring back to the diagram on the next page will help.

Using the Five Aspects to Define the Mind Body Axis

[1] All truth is grounded in duality. All coins have two sides.

Start with the obvious. The coin we're referring to here is us—and the duality we're referring to is the two sides of us, our mind and body. Know we're talking about two of the most argued concepts in all of science and philosophy, including, as I said a moment ago, that some argue there is no such thing as a separate mind.

What did Descartes say about this? Again, it's complicated. Let's start by looking at the two main explanations for how the mind and body could be separate. In the first—substance dualism—the mind and body are two different kinds of matter; two different *substances.* And in the second—property dualism—the mind and body are two different *properties* of the same substance.

A Guide to the Five Aspects
of the Vertical Axis

Pretty much everyone agrees we have a mind and body.

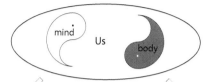

There are two ways to explain it.

dualism

① as Substance Dualism
Our mind and body are two
different kinds of physical
matter.

② as Property Dualism
Our mind and body are two
different properties of the same
kind of matter.

Both these dualisms represent one unity (one "us").

This means there are three ways
to see the mind and body:
[1] as a substance duality
[2] as a property duality
{3] as a unity

③ Simultaneity
Obviously, all three ways of seeing the mind
and body are true. So to know ourselves, we
must somehow keep in mind all three truths.

Doing this is hard.

④ Sums
In theory, we can do this by summing
these three truths. In the real world,
this doesn't work. Because we are
always changing, we are always more
than the sum of these three truths.

⑤ Emergent Properties
Because we are constantly changing,
we are largely chaotic. However, since
fractal patterns always exist within
chaos, by finding these patterns, we
can better our lives.

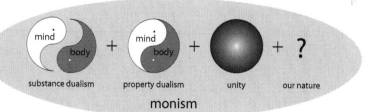

substance dualism   property dualism   unity   our nature

monism

Which side did Descartes take?

He believed in substance dualism, the idea that the mind and body are two entirely different substances. Moreover, Descartes defined the difference between these two substances as that the body has extension, whereas the mind does not.

What is *extension*? Here, we'll stick to the basics. Extension means only that something physically extends out into the physical world—that it takes up space. Obviously, to us, our bodies do and our minds do not.

Know that most people today have trouble understanding how matter could exist without extension, and the reason is simple. Today, we take for granted an alternate explanation—that the opposite of matter is energy.

It was different in Descartes' day. Back then, the concept of *energy* applied only to spiritual things, such as God, goodness, love, and such. So when people began to discover invisible forces—static electricity, centrifugal force, gravity—these forces were seen not as energies but rather, as a special kind of matter; matter-without-extension.

For instance, when William Gilbert introduced the idea of magnetism in 1600 (*On the Magnet and Magnetic Bodies, and on the Great Magnet the Earth*), he described magnetism as *an electric effluvia*. This, he said, was similar in nature to air which is the effluvium in which the earth exists. Moreover, by *effluvium*, he meant an invisible vapor or gas. Thus Gilbert saw magnetism, not as an energy, but rather as an invisible physical substance—as matter-without-extension.

Another example of matter-without-extension was the hypothetical stuff through which light particles were once thought to travel—"luminiferous aether." Quite honestly, I find the arguments as to why we can't see this stuff ingenious. For instance, Isaac Newton proposed that we couldn't see this "aethereal medium" because it transmitted vibrations faster than light (*Opticks*, 1704). Tough to disprove, and logically possible.

These arguments aside, the point is, aethereal aether was considered a substance without extension. Interestingly enough, people argued about this one well into the twentieth century. Moreover, although Aristotle wrote about *energy* in the 4th century B.C. (*Nicomachean Ethics*, 350 B.C., translated by W. D. Ross, Oxford, Clarendon Press, 1908), it wasn't until 1807 that the word *energy* appeared in the modern "qualitative" sense. After which, we began to call matter-without-extension, *energy*.

Does it makes sense now why Descartes called the mind, matter-without-extension? He was merely voicing his ideas in the language of his day. Thus, when he tells us, the mind affects the body and vice versa, he's merely saying that energy affects matter, and vice versa. Not too much of a stretch when you realize what he meant.

— Descartes' Two Substances as the Two-Sides View

Why go through the trouble to point out that "matter-without-extension" is an out-of-date way to refer to energy? Because in order to understand the vertical axis, you must understand why you experience your mind and body as being separate. Here, there are two possibilities. One, you see them as separate because they are made of two kinds of matter. Two, you see them as separate because there are two ways you can define matter—by saying what it is, and by saying what it does—by calling it a substance or by calling it a property.

Today physicists ridicule the first possibility and embrace the second. They tell us that *position* defines matter, and that *momentum* defines energy. In truth though, this difference is more philosophy than science. Rarely will you hear a physicist refer to this as a philosophical distinction though.

Ironically, in Descartes' time, thinking philosophically was an inherent part of being a physicist. Indeed, Descartes called himself a "natural philosopher"—a philosopher of natural phenomena. For centuries, then, the four wise men waged war with each other over this territory, until at last they argued this profession out of existence. At which point, two of them managed to divide up this territory. Which is why today, we see two professions (science and philosophy) where there once was only one.

The thing to see here is where the dividing line exists between these professions. It exists on the vertical axis between the mind and body. And on the body side of the split, we find the materialist wise man's supporters—the physical physicists. They see everything as matter affecting matter. Whereas on the mind side, we find the rationalist wise man's fanboys—the philosophical physicists. They see everything as energies affecting matter.

Overwhelming, isn't it? And we've barely begun to discuss the vertical axis. Are you beginning to see why most folks avoid serious discussions about this stuff. Moreover, it's easy to see why so many scientific types ridicule those who do discuss this stuff. To them, it's just philosophy. Nothing more.

So is it? This is the question raised by the first aspect of the vertical axis. What is the mind made of, matter or energy? Descartes' answer was that the mind is made of a kind of matter, specifically, matter that takes up no space—matter-without-extension. This pleases the materialist wise man, as it makes the mind and body two dissimilar substances. Moreover, because psychophysics appears to support this belief, it's easy to see why

Descartes saw the mind this way. As well as why a twentieth century idea—the physicist's concept of energy—killed this belief.

At the same time, $e=mc^2$ says matter and energy are equivalents, two different forms of the same thing. Thus unless Einstein is wrong, it's obvious, matter and energy do follow the same set of laws, at least at the scale of bodies and planets and solar systems.

So does this mean Descartes is right—that the mind is a different kind of matter? Or is the mind not matter at all, but rather, an energy? When you understand the vertical axis, you know the answer. It's both.

Translating this into everyday language, this means matter and energy are just two ways to refer to the same nameless, universal stuff. This nullifies most of the wise men's arguments and makes the differences between matter-without-extension and energy mere semantics.

— Matter and Energy as Descartes' Two Substances

So what do you think? Was Descartes crazy for thinking the mind is made of an invisible, physical substance? If this is you, then realize that even today, we continue to speak about energies, at times, as if they are invisible substances. For instance, we sometimes talk about how much love we have to give, or how much effort we've made, or how much time we've spent. "How much" is a quality of substances. Yet love, effort, and time are not substances. They're either feelings or ideas, both of which must be energies. Neither is physical, remember?

Where does this leave us? With the idea that one way to experience the difference between the mind and body is to see these two things as the first aspect of the vertical axis describes them—as two different substances. However, to properly understand this axis, we must also look at the other possibility—the idea of property dualism. Here, the mind and body (and matter and energy) are two distinct properties of the same unnamed stuff. This brings us to the second of the five aspects, the rationalist wise man's favorite—*unity*. Know this word is about as close as we come to naming the unnameable stuff.

[2] All duality stems from a unity. Thus while all coins do indeed have two sides, all coins are simultaneously a single object.

Now let's look at the other kind of dualism—property dualism. Know that despite calling this a *dualism*, the focus here is actually on a unity—us—as individual beings. At the same time, this unity—us—has two clearly opposite and distinctly different properties; the mind and the body. Moreover, these two properties are an obvious parallel to the way we see our universe, as a unity—one place—having two clearly opposite and distinctly different sets of properties; matter and energy. Hence the commonly expressed parallels, body to matter and mind to energy.

By inference then, general relativity also supports the second of the five aspects of personal truth—the idea that the mind is in no way a separate substance. Rather, the body and mind, and matter and energy, both arise from the same unnameable, universal stuff. We then experience this nameless universal stuff in two distinctly separate ways—one, as a body with all the properties of material substances, including that they take up space—and two, as a mind with all the properties of non material forces, including that they take up no physical space.

The thing to notice of course is that, in this way of thinking, our mind and body stem from two distinct *experiences*, not from two different *substances*. Here, mind and body are the two ways we experience life. In one, we experience things with extension. In the other, we do not. And both experiences emerge from our interactions with the same nameless, universal stuff.

— Property Dualism (and Spiritual Unity) as the One-Coin View

Here again, we find parallels to what's been said in spiritual belief systems. For instance, in the Tai Chi Tu, everything that exists emerges from one primordial "something," an ineffable all—a unity—represented by the circle. Two complementary properties then emerge from this unity—*yang*, which represents the properties of hot, the heavens, being assertive, the mind, and energy—and *yin*, which represents the properties of cold, the earth, being receptive, the body, and matter.

This viewpoint is clearly stated in the Tao Te Ching. For instance, in Stephen Mitchell's interpretation of verse 42 of the Tao Te Ching (Harper Collins, New York, 1988), he writes:

The Tao gives birth to One.
One gives birth to Two.
Two gives birth to Three.
Three gives birth to all things.

Here, the first two lines describe perfectly the nature of the vertical axis—as a single axis with two sets of opposite properties. Similarly, the vertical axis describes us perfectly as well—as one person with two ways to experience life. First, we experience it from the viewpoint of a body, and second, from the viewpoint of a mind.

Indeed, if you were to read the Gia-Fu Feng / Jane English translation of the Tao Te Ching (Vintage Books, New York, 1989), you'd find they even use the language we've been using here.

The Way gave birth to unity,
Unity gave birth to duality,
Duality gave birth to trinity,
Trinity gave birth to the myriad creatures.

The ten thousand things carry yin and embrace yang.
They achieve harmony by combining these forces.
- Tao Te Ching, Lao Tzu, # 42, c. 500 B.C.

This then is how the second aspect of the vertical axis describes the mind and body—as a unity of two opposite properties, both born of the same nameless, universal stuff.

[3] **To arrive at personal truth, we must keep in mind both the unity and the duality. All coins are simultaneously one coin with two sides.**

So which dualism more accurately describes our mind and body—substance dualism, or property dualism? Or perhaps, the unity of both is the truth? By now, I hope the answer is beginning to be apparent. All three viewpoints describe us accurately. In theory, the mind's truth plus the body's truth equals the whole truth. Here, substance dualism plus the unity of both types of matter are the truth. Whereas in the real world, the mind-body-continuum of truth equals the whole truth. Here, property dualism plus the unity of matter and energy are the truth. And third, the combination of both these things is the whole truth.

Voicing this in the language of the horizontal axis, in theory, each of us is made up of two separate substances—one with, and one without, extension. Thus, in theory, we can be defined by the unity which encompasses this pair of opposites. However, in the real world, we are made up of only one kind of stuff. But this stuff exhibits two clearly opposite and distinctly different properties—the properties of yang, energy, and the mind, and the properties of yin, matter, and the body. Thus in the real world, we can be defined by a unity of all these properties taken separately and together.

— Reconciling the Three Views as One Coin with Two Sides

How do we reconcile these differing views? This is what the third aspect explains. Moreover, if you follow the diagram on the next page, this will go easier.

First we create a continuum from these two dualisms. Then we juxtapose this continuum with a unity containing both. Know that this figure—which is called, a tritinuum—is one of the ways the wise men

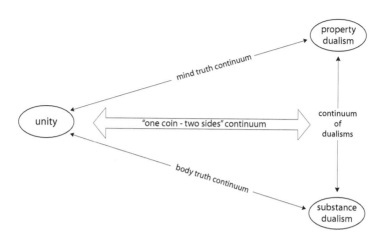

find truth. You'll learn a lot about how to use this shape to find truth in Book III.

For now, the thing to focus on is what we get by using this shape. We get the "one coin with two sides" view. Here, either substance dualism or property dualism is true on one end, and a blend of both dualities is true on the other. Hence the "one coin with two sides" view. Truth is either, or both.

—The One-Coin-with-Two-Sides View as Monism

What do all these mental gymnastics accomplish?

By including both types of dualism, we honor the nature of our world. In this view, the *two sides* view, the world is comprised of pairs of opposites, e.g. yin and yang, body and mind, matter and energy. And by juxtaposing this continuum of dualisms to the unity of both, we then create an alternate view of our world. In this view, the *one coin* view, there is no separation. Everything is connected to everything else.

Know this particular tritinuum has a name. It's called *monism*. And it's considered to be dualism's philosophical opposite. Which means what exactly? Remember the universal nameless stuff I've been speaking about? Monists believe the world consists of varying forms of this nameless, universal stuff. For some, this stuff is called God. For others, it's called nature. And for others, it is simply the entirety of the physical world.

Whatever the case, to monists, nothing can be separate, including the mind and body. Either the body is the whole truth and the mind just a neurochemical illusion—a kind of biological slight of hand trick which gives us a survival advantage. Or the mind is the only true reality and the body, an experiential manifestation of this true reality—the "everything is made of energy" point of view.

Are the monists right? Indeed they are. At the same time, so are both camps of dualists. Moreover, if, at this point, your head feels like it is about to split in two, don't feel too bad. Some of the biggest brains on our planet have been wrestling with these questions—and arguing over these terms—for millennia now. Not coincidentally, Descartes and I are both in this group. Perhaps this explains why our hat sizes are abnormally large?

The thing is, if you understand the vertical axis, you understand what makes answering these questions hard. It states that to find personal truth, you must simultaneously be aware of the unity and both dualities, the one-coin view and the two-sides views.

So is doing this difficult? Duh! Does a bear do its business in the woods? Yes, it's difficult. In fact, in the real world, it's literally impossible. Fortunately for us, the fourth aspect cuts us some slack. In the process, it also explains what it means to be human.

[4] In theory, we can sum these three truths. In the real world, we cannot. Thus personal truths are always more than the sum of the prior three aspects.

If, at this point, you've even marginally followed all this heady stuff, then please give yourself a hearty pat on the back. You certainly deserve it. If, on the other hand, you're starting to feel like a deer in the headlights, don't despair. You haven't entered the Twilight Zone, and you're still perfectly normal. You just lack ways to picture these ideas. That's all.

This brings us to the fourth aspect of personal truth, the aspect which explains why finding these pictures is so hard. It states, in theory, if we sum the first three aspects of the vertical axis, we'll know everything there is to know about the mind and body. However, in the real world—where truth is always more than the sum of the parts—there will always be things about the mind and body we can't know.

In theory then, the diagram on the prior page contains everything there is to know about the mind and body—[1] that the mind and body are two substances, [2] that the mind and body are two properties of one substance, and [3] that if you take these two substances and two properties and juxtapose them to a single self which contains them both, you end up with a closed triad of continuums which describes the complete mind body enchilada.

Unfortunately, in the real world, we can't fully grasp any of these ideas. Trying to read the past few pages should be enough to tell you that. So what can we do?

We can remember Bacon and Descartes. And if we take our lead from Descartes, we can take encouragement from knowing that we may someday know the whole mind body thing. At least, in theory. Yea. At the same time, if we take our lead from Bacon, we can let ourselves off the hook for not knowing it all, as in the real world, nothing can be known entirely.

What amazes me about these two positions is that so many people find Descartes' advice desirable and Bacon's advice hard to take. To wit, many folks spend more time arguing whether the dualism exists than they do using what they know to seek personal truth. The arguments? If both mind and body exist, then how do they interact or coexist? And if they don't, then what are we experiencing when we think and or feel?

Fortunately, this is one of the mysteries the wise men's map explains. In the next chapter, I'll show you how. For now, all you need know is that you need not take sides to solve this mystery. You need only acknowledge that all parties are right. But only in their own realms and in relation to each other.

The problem, of course, is that we're still left with the same dilemma Bacon faced. Despite being able to see the logical truth in all this beautiful theory, in the real world, we have no way to conclusively prove any of it. However, as I told you a moment ago, this dilemma exists only because it's hard to picture these ideas, that's all. And in the next chapter, I'll not only give you a way to picture these ideas. I'll also reveal what's prevented us from solving this mystery.

— Pictures as a Way to Understand the Fourth Aspect

Finally, with regard to how the fourth aspect defines the mind and body, the thing to remember is this. In theory, we can know all there is to know about the mind and body. Theoretical wholes equal the sum of the parts. But since theories are ideas and as such, do not exist physically, theoretical wholes cannot be pictured, except symbolically.

At the same time, because real world wholes do exist physically, real world wholes can be pictured. So although, on paper, they're nightmarishly complex, we can, after all, see real world things, including ourselves.

My point is, please don't worry if you haven't understood what's been said here. The technical side of the fourth aspect simply says that real world wholes equal the sum of the parts plus some unknowable nature. In terms of the mind and body, this means we are each a mind plus a body plus the nature of this unity. Moreover, all you need to take away from this dreadful mess of words that we can't put the entirety of who we are down on paper.

More important, it does not say we can't know ourselves. Only that we can't put it into words. Indeed, the most important thing the fourth aspect has to teach us is that there is a way for us to see real world sums, including the sum of our mind and body—our personal truth. To do this, we need to use pictures. This is it. And no, we'll never know ourselves or anyone else completely. But if we use pictures, we can get close enough to use what we can know to better our lives.

Here then lies the path to your personal truth. If you can picture something, you can interact with it, and if you keep on trying, you can make changes. So while in theory, it's tough to know yourself because you can't picture theories, in the real world, you can picture yourself. Thus as counterintuitive as it may sound, coming to know yourself in the real world is infinitely easier than knowing yourself in theory, even if the real world you is infinitely complex.

[5] The idea of emergent properties explains why we can't sum these ideas to find personal truth. The nature of real world things exists only when they are in their natural state. This makes personal truth an emergent quality of the simultaneously-experienced combination of theoretical world truth plus real world truth.

Boiling what we've just said down to its essence then, it's obvious what the fifth aspect has to tell us about the mind and body. Like all things in the real world, our mind and body constantly change. Moreover, since we are the living combination of this mind and body, our overall nature is constantly emerging as well.

In other words, since change is the fundamental constant underlying all naturally occurring things, our nature is constantly being reinvented. This makes real world things, like you and I, infinitely complex, and renders any and all attempts to know ourselves, either by direct measurement or by summing the parts, doomed from the start.

So does this mean we can never truly know ourselves?

Theorists and real worlders alike refuse to accept this. And I applaud them for doing this. Like Socrates said, the unexamined life is not worth living. Moreover, while both groups acknowledge how complex human beings are, they each believe they have a way around this—theorists by reducing the mind and body to intellectually analyzable parts and logically knowable ideas—real worlders by pragmatically separating the mind and body into categories of knowable physiology and observable behavior.

The problem, of course, with both these methods is that they deny the need for the other. Thus by inference, both theorists and real worlders alike believe you can dissect a human being into more manageable parts, then know this being by measuring then summing these parts. This is like trying to know a pie by baking it one ingredient at a time, then trying to reassemble these baked ingredients into an edible pie. It can't be done. Just as you can't take a pie out of the oven before it's done and know how it will turn out either. Yet these kinds of things are exactly what theorists and real worlders alike attempt to do when they extract real world things, like human beings, from their environment, then try to reduce them to their constituent parts, thinking they can know the nature of a person by summing these parts.

Strangely, this is one of the things the overzealous watchdogs of science frequently fail to account for. These folks claim we can find truth only by following strictly scientific protocols. Yet in reality, these protocols can never reveal the whole truth, as dividing any real world thing into parts changes its nature, even atoms.

This means any scientist who claims these sums are a whole truth is a poor scientist indeed, a conclusion natural philosophers knew centuries ago. At the same time, failing to see the good in reductionism is just as foolish. Part to wholes—whole to parts—both offer truth.

— Descartes as the Advocate of Fractals

What about Descartes? Didn't he urge us to divide things into parts? Admittedly, a literal read of Descartes' method does seem to imply he believed we could and should do this. The thing is, if you read the man in his own words, you find something most folks overlook. On the way to writing his *Discourse on Method*, Descartes wrote the rather detailed and unfortunately unfinished treatise I mentioned previously—*Rules For the Direction of the Mind*. In it, Descartes outlines his intention to put into words what to me would have been the most amazing part of his method. Descartes refers to fractals. Not in so many words, mind you. The word didn't exist until the late twentieth century. Still, the concept is there if you know what to look for—Descartes' admission that we must address non linear things.

In addition, if you overlook Descartes' first step and begin at his second, he does indeed advise us to divide what we're exploring into parts. However, his first step tells we must start with a unity—with intuition—a concept he later disguises as logic by calling it, "intuitive reasoning" (*Meditations*, 1641, response to Antoine Arnauld).

What does all this mean? Simply this. If you ignore Descartes' first step, you've taken Descartes' method out of context. Thus while many folks are quick to quote the second step, rarely do they point to what precedes it as anything useful, let alone important. Yet Descartes himself tells us intuition is the whole from which the parts emerge, and that for us to find our truth, we must see both the whole and the parts.

— The Two Conclusions We Can Draw From the Fifth Aspect

Descartes aside, the point is, the fifth aspect tells us two things about the mind and body. One, that the infinite complexity of us as wholes can't be put down on paper—and two, that we can't divide ourselves into a mind and body, then know ourselves by summing what we find.

Where does this leave us? To be honest, with a lot of hope. The fifth aspects tells us we can indeed know ourselves, this despite the ever-present chaos. How? By using fractals to discern between what is and isn't knowable.

What isn't knowable? The sum of anything chaotic. And since the nature of real things includes constant change—and since the nature of this constant change is that it is, in part, chaotic—sums cannot predict the nature of anything real, including us.

At the same time, by inference, this defines for us what is knowable about ourselves. Not directly. Not in so many words. But it's inferred by the idea which underlies this chaos—the idea of constant change.

How can you know the nature of something which constantly changes? It's simple. You forget about trying to add it up and focus entirely on the patterns in this change. Or in Descartes' sense of the words, you see the chaos of intuition as the primordial ooze out of which these knowable patterns of change emerge.

Know these patterns exist even when you cannot see them—in things like hurricanes, and snow storms, and rain clouds. So yes, things like weather change constantly, making predicting the weather near impossible. But even within the chaos of weather, there are changes which can be predicted—the nature of rain clouds after they form, the nature of snow storms after they begin, even the nature of hurricanes once they appear.

Applying this idea to us as living beings, this means there are knowable patterns within our personalities, organic fractals which apply to all of us. Know I'm not referring here to anything like cultural habits or social norms. I'm referring to discernible, universal patterns of mind body interactions. And yes, like all fractals, these universal patterns of human behavior and experience manifest in infinitely complex ways. At the same time, once they begin, these patterns are as recognizable to us as rain clouds (grief and sadness), and snow storms (passive aggression and apathy), and hurricanes (anger and arguments).

How Does This Help Us Find Our Truth?

What have we gained from applying the five aspects to the vertical axis? Are we any closer to our truth? Indeed, we are. We now have a way to honor all four wise men's truths, both in our mind and in our body. To do this, we must first discern between what we can and cannot know. We must then look for the fractal patterns present in what we can know, and when we find them, we've found our truth.

How does one go about finding these fractal patterns? This is what I'll be teaching you in the rest of this series. In Book II, I'll show you how to find the patterns in Personality. In Book III, I'll show you how to find the patterns in the rest of the universe. And in both books, we'll focus on finding patterns in the chaos.

For now, you might want to take a break though. This stuff can be hard to read. Hell. Can be? It is hard. In fact, I strongly urge you to take a break. Go screw off for a few days. Or more, even. And yes, I realize that much of what you've just been through may have felt like a cross between your first piano lessons and learning the times tables. However, if you stick it out, I promise, you'll learn some really amazing stuff. For one thing, how to have your own original ideas.

My point? Hang in there. This chapter is the worst of it. The series gets easier as it goes on.

The Axis Mundi (the seat of the fifth wise man)

Now we come to the part of the map at the heart of the action, the Axis Mundi. So let me ask you. Have you heard this phrase before? You may have. It's as old as the Tao symbol. Some say older. The term itself is Latin and literally means, "center of the world." And while many cultures have their own names for this ubiquitous symbol—the world pillar, the navel of the world, the Bodhi Tree, the cosmic axis—what it represents is always the same. It's the place to which a seeker must travel to find his or her truth.

This then is the first thing to know about the Axis Mundi. Like most of the ideas in this book, this one is not new either. Every culture has stories wherein a shaman, priestess, hero, or adventurer makes a journey to the Axis Mundi, always for the same purpose—to find his or her truth.

Where is the center of the world located? Tradition tells us it exists at the intersection of the four compass directions, on a vertical path between the sky and the earth. But where exactly is this intersection point?

Usually it's been said to exist far from the normal world, often at some high, difficult to reach place. For instance, in Japan, it was said to be located on Mount Fuji. For the ancient Greeks, it was located on the southwestern spur of Mount Parnassus in the valley of Phocis at Delphi. For the Sioux, it was located in the Black Hills. For the Australian Pitjantjatjara people, it was located at Uluru, a large sandstone rock formation in the southern part of the Northern Territory, central Australia. And for the Taoists, it was located at Mount Kun-Lun, the great mountain system of central Asia between the Himalayas and the Tian Shan. No coincidence, they called this mountain, the mountain "at the middle of the world."

Sometimes, too, people claimed the Axis Mundi was a man-made place. For instance, in ancient Mesopotamia, the Sumerians and Babylonians erected artificial mountains called *ziggurats,* and these were seen as the Axis Mundi. Similarly, for the pre-Columbian Mayans, the pyramids of Teotihuacán in Mexico were the Axis Mundi. And for the ancient Egyptians, the pyramids at Giza were the Axis Mundi.

As for the wise men, they say the Axis Mundi lies at the intersection of their four realms. Indeed, there is even a tradition that supports this idea. That it is probably one of the oldest Axis Mundi traditions only adds to its significance. Here we're talking about The Garden of Eden, out of which the four sacred rivers were said to flow. And at the center of this garden was said to be the Tree of Knowledge of Good and Evil, yet another reference to the place where you must go in order to find your truth.

Of course, the question everyone asks is how the Axis Mundi can be in more than one place? After all, by definition, wouldn't there be only one center of the world? Here, I'll defer to the wisdom of the Buddhists who say the Axis Mundi is not a physical place. Rather it exists beneath you, wherever you are. And yes, they teach that the Buddha found enlightenment while sitting under the Bodhi Tree. But they also teach that the Bodhi Tree exists wherever you sit your practice.

This then is where you'll find your Axis Mundi. It lies at the center of wherever you are, right beneath you. Moreover, if you can visualize the four compass points and a vertical path between the sky and the earth intersecting these four points, you'll have an even better shot at finding your truth. Considering we live in such a busy world, it's also quite convenient. Your personal truth comes with you wherever you go.

Most important of all though is knowing what sitting in this seat will do for you. You can know by what this seat is called. It's called the seat of the fifth wise man. (Or wise woman, if you prefer.) And who exactly is this fifth wise man? Why it's you, of course, whenever you chose to sit in this seat.

This makes the four wise men's Axis Mundi sort of a cross between a metaphysical Switzerland and The Land of Oz. Like Switzerland, it's located on neutral ground in the center of the four realms—the East, West, North, and South. And like the Emerald City in the Land of Oz—wherein four lands are ruled by one monarch—it is the place to which the hero makes his journey, the wise man finds his wisdom, the spiritual guide, her purpose, and the saint, her personal faith.

Does what I've been telling you sound like nonsense? Then try reading anything on mythic heroes, ancient or modern, Joseph Campbell's *The Hero with a Thousand Faces* (Princeton University Press, 1972), for instance, or Clarissa Pinkola Estes' *Women Who Run with the Wolves* (Ballantine Books, 1992). If you do, you'll find that these stories have existed throughout history, from Jacob's Ladder and Jack and the Beanstalk to Odin and the World Ash Tree. Even the Arthur legends and the story of Rapunzel describe this hero's journey. As does Dante Alighieri's *The Divine Comedy*.

And if the rationalist wise man is your hero, meaning, if you feel you are too intelligent to believe in this kind of stuff? All I can say is that you might want to spend some time researching the lives of the great men and women in science. In every case, you'll find something which functioned as the Axis Mundi, often the belief that if you can find the starting point from which to discover a truth, that you can bring this wisdom back to the world and make it a better place.

How Can Facts and Ideas Only Be True in Theory?

Before I close this chapter, I need to clear up a few things. Specifically, the idea that some things are true only in theory. In other words, if you look at the map of the wise men's realms, you'll see that two of the four great truths—facts and ideas—don't exist in the real world. They exist only in theory. But if this is so, then why do we treat facts and ideas as if they can exist in the real world?

Let's start with the materialist wise man's truth—facts. How can I seriously be saying that facts don't exist in the real world?

One thing which makes me say this is the idea that all facts occur in frozen moments. This is the first criteria for a fact—a fixed moment in time. In other words, to get a fact, we must make a measurement—and to make a measurement, we must stop a clock. In the real world, though, we can't stop a clock. So the best we can say is that, in theory, this fact was once true in the real world. It was true in that theoretically frozen moment in time.

Why then do we stubbornly adhere to the belief that facts are real world truths? Because if they were, we could, in theory, predict the future. And prevent many problems. Indeed, this desire to predict the future is what underlies Einstein' refusal to believe in the uncertainty principle. If facts don't exist in the real world, then there is much about life we can never control. An unsettling thought for all of us, but especially for a physicist.

What about statistical measurements? Can't we use statistics to derive measurements which function almost as well as facts?

In theory, we can. This is why we use statistical trends to guide our decisions. But this method has limits. Statistics treat time averaged as a valid substitute for the present moment. Thus even the most naive among us know statistical truths aren't the same as real world truths.

How do we attempt to compensate for this limit? We retest things, again and again. We do this, assuming, if our results stay the same, we can statistically average these results, then treat them as real world facts.

Is retesting a valid way to derive facts though? In other words, is there a point at which we can say that observing the same outcome makes a fact, a real world truth? Well, let's look. Say we're talking about the winner of a horse race. We call this winner, a fact. And in theory, this is correct. But were we to rerun this horse race two minutes later and if the same horse won, would this prove this horse would always be the winner? Obviously, not.

What if we reran the race a third time, and a fourth time, and a fifth, and what if the same horse won? Would this prove this fact existed in the real world? Obviously, not. This is why we qualify things like horse race winners by calling them *historical* facts. To the best of our knowledge, at this moment in history, this outcome *was*, not is, a fact.

This then is the reason facts can't exist in the real world. All facts are historical facts. In other words, facts exist only in fixed moments in the past. Thus, while they may have once measured something pretty accurately, now, they no longer do. And while, in theory, we can stop a clock and get a fact anytime we want, in the real world, time waits for no wise man.

Overall then, the thing to keep in mind about facts being true in the real world is this. Despite the materialist wise man's claim that facts are the only reliable truth, in the real world, we cannot know. Maybe we measured them accurately. Maybe we made a mistake. But whatever the case, because all facts—including scientific facts—exist only in the past, we can never claim they are real world truths. Yet another example of Descartes' knowable unknowable thing.

So much for predicting the future.

How Change is What Makes Real World Things Real

Does what I've just said sound crazy? Then let me try a different tact, this time, with the focus on the second core quality of facts—physical position. What I mean is, as I've defined them, to have a fact you must have three things—a fixed time, a fixed place, and a single, precise measurement. And in theory, we can do all three. But in the real world, we can meet only one of these criteria. Indeed, this problem is what the famous Greek philosopher, Parmenides, and his contemporary, Heraclitus, argued about.

To Parmenides, change is an illusion, and truth is timeless and uniform. And in theory, he's right. But when Heraclitus proclaimed, "you cannot step into the same river twice," he was right too. Thus a good way to see why facts can't be real world truths is that nothing stands still. Except in theory.

What about the other theoretical truth—ideas? Can ideas exist in the real world? Here these same criteria—time and position—apply. Thus with ideas, time is eternal, and ideas hold true regardless of where you state them. So are ideas real? Again, we'll turn to our two Greek philosophers, Parmenides and Heraclitus, for answers.

According to Parmenides, nothing other than appearances change. Ideas are truly eternal and equally true no matter where or when you state them. According to Heraclitus though, "we both step and do not step in the same rivers. We are and are not." (Diels, Hermann Alexander. (1879) *Doxographi Graeci.* Berlin). Thus, Heraclitus agrees with Descartes. We can either know something as true, or know we cannot know.

How do the two real world truths apply to facts and ideas? For instance, do your feelings about facts and ideas change?

Indeed, they do. Feelings are a real world truth, and all real world truths change constantly. So, too, will any stories you may tell regarding how you came to observe this fact or know this idea. Each time you tell these stories, or relate this idea, something will change, even if only by emphasis. And since facts, and ideas, by definition, do not change, neither feelings nor stories can be part of what makes a fact or an idea true.

This, then, is the best way to see how something can be true "only in theory." *Change is what makes real world things real.* Conversely, the lack of change is what makes theoretical things true. For instance, in the real world, a river can't stand still. However, in theory, we can never know. Indeed, were we to continue to follow this question down the imaginary rabbit hole, we could get lost in it. Can we theoretically step into the same river twice? How about three times or more? In theory, yes, we can. As many times as we want. Step lively now. But only in theory.

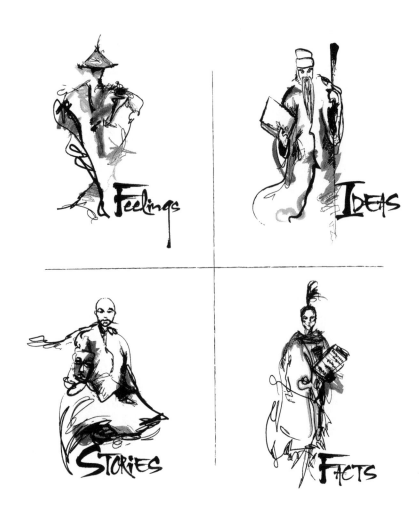

Notes Written in the Margins of Chapter Three

On the Origin of the Word *Theory*

Years ago, when I was even more arrogant, I overheard two young medical doctors talking about how they were going to teach something. At the time I was eating in a local breakfast cafe, and they were sitting at the next table. A discussion ensued in which I tried, to no avail, to explain how picturing was the key to understanding. At which point, the second in command, commenting on my theory, asked me if I knew the origin of the word *theory*. Despite being a young know-it-all, somehow, I didn't. At which point, he related this story.

In ancient Greece, medical doctors trained in amphitheaters. Real amphitheaters, of course. Here, the operation would occur in the middle of this amphitheater and the student doctors would sit at ground level so they could be close to what was going on. The oldest and most experienced doctors would then sit in the highest seats. And while they'd be farther away from the action, they'd have the best overview.

These seats were called the *theoria*.

Can you see how nicely this explains the physical placement of the rationalist wise man's realm?

On the Existence of *Aether*

Despite the fact that we claim to have disproved the existence of "aether" early in the twentieth century, recent discoveries point to that there may well be a modern equivalent called *dark matter*. Here, the word *dark* refers to that we cannot see this stuff, as in it remains in the dark. Amazingly, physicists tell us that visible matter accounts for only 1% of the matter in our universe. And while they think they can account for about 10% of the invisible stuff, they haven't a clue as to how to account for the rest.

Invisible matter. Dark matter. Are you getting this? Perhaps they should just give in and call it *aether*? Or at least, *matter without extension*?

On the Words *Matter* and *Energy*

One of the most amazing things about language is how it gives us insight into how our minds work, especially with regard to how we think our world works. Take the word *reify*. Do you know this word? In case you don't, it means *to treat the idea of something as if it had concrete or material existence*. I raise this because this word holds the key to understanding terms like matter and energy. In other words, to be blunt, while there is indeed a Santa Claus, there is no such thing as matter or energy. These two words—and the concepts they represent—are entirely made up.

Most folks don't know this though, including most physicists. They treat these two concepts as if they are literal, hold 'em in your hand, things. Yet if you boil down substance dualism and property dualism to their essence, you find energy and matter are just different ways to refer to the same nameless stuff. In one, we have invisible matter which affects things. In the other, we have invisible energy which affects things.

The thing to notice of course is how valuable the word *reify* can be when it comes to discerning personal truth. And if you combine this concept with the equals sign, you end up flushing a whole lot of mind poop right down the porcelain disposal unit. To wit, what the heck do you think $e=mc^2$ means anyway? Physicists tell us it means energy equals mass times the speed of light squared. And this means what exactly? That mass times the speed of light squared, which we normal folks call *matter*, equals energy.

Now at this point, I feel I should apologize to those physicists who either know this as true and should by rights be called natural philosophers, or those who would point out all the wonderfully complex and enormously important understandings we can and do derive if we use these two concepts.

My point is, please don't get too hung up on getting a physicist's understanding of the things I'm telling you. Plain old everyday understandings and common sense often lead to more personal truth than the most obtuse of technical formulas. And if you're still missing my point, consider what professor Don Howard of the University of Notre Dame has to say about Einstein:

One of the secrets to Einstein's success was that he was well read in philosophy, and that guided his approach not only to framing and solving problems in physics but also to interpreting his discoveries in a more universal context. In addition, his philosophy background gave him the independence of judgment necessary to invent a new physics (Albert Einstein: Physicist, Philosopher, and Humanitarian, The Teaching Company, Course 8122, Chantilly, VA, 2008).

Gee, does this sound like Einstein was a natural philosopher? Today's physicists might be surprised to know that all the great physicists were, ancient and modern alike. This includes not only Einstein but also people like Richard Feynman, Neils Bohr, Erwin Schrödinger, Werner Heisenberg, and Stephen Hawking. Heisenberg, later in life, even wrote a book titled *Physics and Philosophy*. Feynman attributed much of his success to his father instilling in him a sense of awe and wonder, a comment reminiscent of Aristotle's oft quoted line that *philosophy begins in wonder*. Neils Bohr based his family crest on a symbol taken from Taoist philosophy. And Stephen Hawking had meetings with the Pope to discuss how his work in physics could be reconciled with the teachings of Catholicism.

Resources for Chapter Three—The Wise Men's Map

On The Teaching Company

A moment ago, I quoted from a description of a course being offered by The Teaching Company. You should know, these guys and gals are the real deal. Moreover, while I don't always agree with everything their professors have to say, I so enjoy their stuff and heartily recommend it. And by all means, spring for the video rather than just the audio. Picturing is the key to understanding, remember?

The following were used as background to this chapter:

Howard, Don. (2008). *Albert Einstein: Physicist, Philosopher, and Humanitarian*. Course 8122. Chantilly, VA: The Teaching Company.

Goldman, Steven L. (2006). *Science Wars: What Scientists Know and How They Know It*. Course 1235. Chantilly, VA: The Teaching Company.

Modern Physicists as Natural Philosophers

Heisenberg, Werner. (1958). *Physics and Philosophy. The Revolution in Modern Science*. New York: Harper Collins.

(Toward the end of this book, a young Heisenberg is quoted as saying, in response to advice that he study Einstein and Plank, that he was *much more interested in the underlying philosophical ideas than in the rest*. Duh! Can you say, natural philosopher. He's also quoted as saying that someone complained to him at the 1927 Solvay Conference that Einstein keeps talking about God, wherein someone else answered that Plank was worse in that he sees no contradiction between religion and science. The stories a man tells tell a lot about the man, don't they?)

Capra, Fritjof. (1996). *The Web of Life: A New Understanding of Living Systems*. New York: Anchor Books, Random House Inc.

Capra, Fritjof. (2000, 1975). *The Tao of Physics, An Exploration of the Parallels between Modern Physics and Eastern Mysticism*. Boston: Shambhala Publications.

(Capra is one of the people with whom I've had imaginary conversations. His later book, *The Web of Life*, is among my favorites. Like many geniuses, he's so dense, he's hard to read. Yet he's so real, he's hard not to read. Slowly, of course. Very slowly.)

Feynman, Richard P. (1995). *The Meaning of It All, Thoughts of a Citizen-Scientist*. New York: Basic Books. (Originally this was a three part lecture Feynman gave in 1963. In it, he talks, often irreverently, about a wide variety of topics from the conflict between science and religion to the need to overhaul the English language. Between Feynman, Einstein, Da Vinci, and Frank Zappa, I've come to believe that irreverence is a prerequisite for genius. Hopefully my own irreverence will be seen in this same light some day.)

Bohr, Niels Henrik David. (1987). *Atomic Theory and the Description of Nature (The Philosophical Writings of Niels Bohr)*. Vol. 1 Woodbridge, CT: Ox Bow Press.

(A collection of Bohr's essays written from 1925 to 1962.)

Bohr, Niels Henrik David. (1987). *Essays 1932-1957 on Atomic Physics and Human Knowledge*. Woodbridge, CT: Ox Bow Press.

(A second collection of Bohr's essays. That Bohr included in his design of his family crest the Tao symbol speaks volumes. 'Nuff said.)

Einstein, Albert and Alan Harris. (2006). *The World as I See It (Mein Weltbild)*. New York: Kensington Publishing Corporation.

Einstein, Albert and Carl Seelig. (1995). *Ideas and Opinions*. New York: Crown Publishing Group.

(Need I say anything at all about the man who called God, *the Old One*.)

Hawking, Stephen. (1996). *The Illustrated A Brief History of Time*. New York: Bantam Books.

Hawking, Stephen. (2001, 1996). *The Universe in a Nutshell*. New York: Bantam Books.

(One of the marks of a genius is that his or her work is ridiculed. So when I found an entire book dedicated to making Hawking a pseudo-scientist, I had to laugh. That this book and it's author shall remain unnamed here is the best FU I can give it. Moreover, you don't have to agree with everything Stephen Hawking says to see that he is a man of courage and conviction. I admire him. Those who don't, FU.)

Modern Translations of Ancient Philosophers

Mitchell, Stephen. (2000). *Bhagavad Gita, A New Translation*. New York: Harmony Books.

Mitchell, Stephen. (1988). *Tao Te Ching, A New English Translation*. New York: Harper Collins.

(If your motive is to gain an understanding of what you're reading, Mitchell is outstanding. And yes, he has his biases, as do we all. But when a translator can open your mind and heart to what is being said, this carries far more weight than mere word-perfection. Try reading the preface to his translation of the Bhagavad Gita, for instance. Awesome.)

Feng, Gia-Fu and Jane English. (1989). *Tao Te Ching*. New York: Vintage Books.

Chapter 4

Using Words—Solving the Mind Body Mystery

The Mystery of the Mind Body Connection

In this chapter, we're going to explore what I see as one of the more interesting things in this book—a real answer to the mind body mystery, including that representatives of all four wise men will present evidence for how this pair of opposites can exist. And interact. Being as they've been arguing about these questions for almost four hundred years now, this chapter is bound to cause the stuff to hit the fan. At the same time, when stuff hits the fan, it's often the prelude to self discovery. So if you've been looking to make a major discovery about yourself, I promise, you'll get the chance to do that in this chapter.

What exactly will we be talking about? To start with, I'm going to tell you a bit about how I came to be so interested in this mind body thing. I wasn't always, you know, albeit, like many people, I've wondered about it on and off for much of my life. I've also, at times, asked the same kinds of questions you've probably asked yourself. Do we really have a separate mind and body, or is this just an illusion? If they do exist separately, then do they interact, and if so, how? What about what the mind is made of? Is the mind, the soul? Or is the mind just a sophisticated bio-computer, and how can we know for sure?

The Mind Body Speedometer
(how frequency affects access to the two brains)

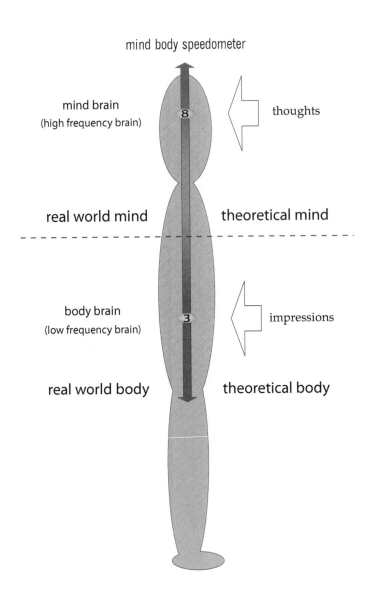

mind body speedometer

mind brain
(high frequency brain)

8

thoughts

real world mind   theoretical mind

body brain
(low frequency brain)

3

impressions

real world body   theoretical body

Of course, were you to ask the four wise men's copywriters, you'd find they all claim to know. For instance, recently, I've noticed a number of books claiming "there is no separate mind—there is no soul—there is no God—it's all just a wicked plot." I've also seen a bunch which blame the evils of the world on the people who write these books. For cripes sake, I've even seen one bashing Descartes, equating his *Discourse on Method* to Hitler's autobiography, *Mein Kamph*. And these are intelligent folks, or at least they seem to be. So why they would prefer to bash others rather than offer real answers is beyond me. Given how the four wise men just love to throw stuff at the fan, I guess I shouldn't be surprised.

Why bring this up? Because to be honest, books which attack a person's character to disprove their theories bother me. To say the least, it's bad science. At its worst, it closes minds. At the same time, as bad as these outbursts are, they sometimes motivate people. In my case, this is exactly what happened. Something about the materialists saying it's stupid to believe in a separate mind just set me off and got me thinking.

Then something strange happened, the kind of thing Carl Jung might have called a "synchronous event." In the same week, two patients whom had never met and didn't know each other raised questions in me as to where they were getting their sense of time from. This led me to wonder where we all get our sense of time from. Do you know? I didn't. Nor did I realize this has been one of our greatest philosophical mysteries. As it turns out, it's also the key to solving the mind body mystery as well.

My question about where people get their sense of time then led me to reread a book called *The Second Brain—Your Gut Has a Mind of Its Own* by Dr. Michael D. Gershon (HarperCollins, New York, 1998). For anyone unfamiliar with Dr. Gershon's work, this book is an interesting read. I also find it to be an example of science at its best—careful, consistent, and free of blame. Despite this, many of Dr. Gershon's peers balk at his use of the word *brain*. Considering how territorial M.D.'s can be, this shouldn't surprise me either. Moreover, these objectors raise a valid point—what makes something a brain? This question turned out to be important as well.

Introducing Dr. Gershon's Two Physiological Brains

Where does Dr. Gershon's work fit into this mind body story?

To start with, his book proves we have two physiological brains—one in the head, and one in the gut. Moreover, there are two things that make me certain he is right in calling them both *brains*. One, both brains can function independently of each other. To wit, if you sever all the nerves which connect the cranial brain and spine to the gut, the gut will still function. And of course, so will the cranial brain. And two, in order for these two brains to be able to function separately, they must each have their own sense of time, a master clock so to speak which, among other things, allows them to interface both with each other and with the rest of the world. Here, by master clock, I'm referring to something which determines when and for how long they do things.

Where do the mind and body come in? It turns out that these two master clocks run at different speeds. Moreover, this gives us two completely different ways to sense time, the mind's way and the body's.

How are they different?

Obviously, the brain in the head, is, by design, more powerful. And the brain in the gut is more primitive. No surprise then that the brain in the head processes time more quickly than the brain in the gut.

More important still is the difference in how these two brains sense time. Thus it turns out, they not only run at different speeds. They also process time differently.

To wit, the brain in our gut gives us *one-moment-at-a-time* time. This happens to be the best way to sense time when you're doing physical things. Focus only on what you're doing now. Whereas, the brain in the head gives us *time-over-time* time. Here you focus not only on what you're doing now, but also on what you've done and what you're about to do. Thus it's from the brain in our head that we get our mental ability to preemptively multitask.

Time-over-time. One-moment-at-a-time. Fast and powerful. Slow and thorough. Basically, this is the main difference between our two brains. Not surprisingly, this difference in large part determines what we will or will not do well. Either we'll be good at planning and being on time, but will struggle to live in the present moment—not enough awareness of the brain in the gut. Or we'll be good at living in the present moment, but suck at planning and being on time—not enough awareness of the brain in the head.

Does this make sense yet? If a brain needs to consider multiple points in time, it has to be powerful. And fast. Otherwise it would constantly lose it's place, and nothing would get done. Conversely, if all a brain needs to do is to deal with one moment in time, it can be much less powerful and still function fine. It should also run much slower, so it can be more focused on what it's doing.

How, then, does this actually affect our lives and who we are?

We each have two sides to our personality, each of these brains contributing half. From our mind's brain we get our belief in cause and effect, our love of logic and reason, and our sense that all things come in pairs of opposites. And from our body's brain we get our belief that we can happily-ever-after, our love of sports, music, and the arts, and our feeling that all things are attributes of the one.

With regard to truth then, to the mind, truth is either a sequence that leads to an idea (that and that caused this to happen) or a sequence of feelings (first I felt this, then I felt that). Whereas to the body, truth is either a single, measured observation, as in one fact (this thing happened), or a single group of measured observations, as in one story (this event happened). And yes, I'm well aware that what I've just said—that the focus in stories is on wholes not sequences of parts, and that the focus in feelings is on sequences of parts not wholes—may have just put a run in your mental pantyhose. If so, don't worry. Before we're done, this will all make sense.

How These Two Brains Explain Who We Are

So let me ask you. Can you see, even at this point, how having two brains would explain a lot about who we are? For instance, do you remember, back in chapter two, we spoke about how experiencing the mind and body separately creates questions in us. For instance, when we feel pain, we look to see where it's coming from, the body or the mind. Having two brains explains why we ask these kinds of questions, and why we tend to feel at times like we're being torn in half inside. And in a real sense, we are, whenever our two brains disagree.

Then there's the way these two brains resemble our two hands. By this, I mean, we all tend to reach with one hand first. We do this with our two brains as well. This leads us to either favor the mind's point of view over the body's as in, *she's so smart, he's such a brute*—or the body's point of view over the mind's as in, *she's an egghead, he's a great athlete*. Moreover, like favoring one hand over the other, favoring one brain over the other affects everything we do, from who we vote for (*experience versus youth*) and which career we choose (*teacher or writer versus doctor or cop*), to who we marry (*intelligent versus wealthy*) and what we eat (*healthy versus fresh*).

In addition, do you remember all the stuff we spoke about back in chapter two regarding the mystery of the *self*? Deep stuff, eh? Having two brains explains why we experience these various selves, as well as why we sometimes lose our sense of having a separate self and selflessly merge with others.

It also explains why our deepest philosophies and religions, all, in their own way, include both the mind body split and the mind body unity. After all, one brain is literally divided into two halves, while the other is not.

Of course, what most folks will find more interesting is how having two brains explains our vulnerabilities to everything from addictions and overeating to Asperger's and ADHD, as well as what this has to tell us about why some of us struggle with managing our money, being on time, being creative, and being able to relax. This two brains thing sure does affect a lot, doesn't it? And if you're beginning to feel overwhelmed by all the possible implications, then consider this. We've been looking for solutions to the mind body mystery for hundreds of years now. Intuitively, we've known it's important. But I expect to be integrating what I've discovered here for the rest of my life. So please don't expect yourself to absorb all this overnight.

One last thing. If you're feeling at all worried that I might, at some point, tell you I've been channeling this stuff from the bowels of a ten-thousand-year-old ascended master, then you should know this. Before the end of this chapter, you'll know for yourself how to test for this two brains thing, empirically, in two minutes or less. It's this obvious. The question this raises of course is, if two minutes is all it takes, then how can we have overlooked something this obvious?

In part, the answer is a no-brainer—it has been hiding in plain sight. But it probably has more to do with what happens to any professional who tries to raise this topic. You've seen it. There's a bloodbath. And it's no wonder. Change what you believe about the mind body interaction and not one of your beliefs would be unaffected. Not about medicine. Not about education. Not about career. Not about family. In truth, nothing in your life would ever be the same. Can you think of anything more scary? Or exciting?

The Four Wise Men's Take On The Mind Body Mystery

Speaking of bloodbaths and changing our beliefs, this brings us to the next thing we'll be looking at in this chapter—the four wise men's views on why we experience the mind and body separately. And how they can interact. Here we'll move our focus away from the physiological aspects of the mind body mystery and onto the psychological aspects. Why haven't we been able to agree on why we experience a separate mind and body? You're about to find out.

Who will present these four views? Four natural philosophers, three of whom you'll likely recognize by name. Know that each of these men personally experienced bloodbaths during his lifetime, in part, for the very ideas they're about to share with you. So while you may disagree with them and think them crazy, you can't say they're not qualified.

Who are these four men anyway? First up is someone I consider to be one of the most misunderstood people in all of history, René Descartes. He'll be representing the materialist wise man. Admittedly, to some, this choice will seem odd. The world considers Descartes to be a rationalist—a man of reason. However, as we learned in the previous chapter, Descartes was also a "substance" dualist. He literally wrote the book on how the mind and body are made of two different kinds of matter. And since what matters most to the materialist wise man is whether the mind and body actually exist, Descartes will defend this view. After all, no sense having this discussion if dualism has no basis in material reality.

Next up will be another thoroughly misunderstood fellow, Baruch de Spinoza, who will represent the spiritual wise man. Here again, this choice may seem odd. After all, Spinoza is also known to the world as a rationalist. The thing is, his pantheistic philosophy is so biased toward the spiritual wise man that it was said to have appalled our next presenter. Pantheism is a form of monism wherein everything in the world is God. Thus Spinoza literally defined substance as *Deus sive natura*—as one and the same thing as God. Ergo, he'll be defending the spiritual wise man's position—that mind and body are the two viewpoints from which we can experience life.

Our third man, Gottfried Wilhelm von Leibnitz, is considered a rationalist as well. However, he too has been reassigned. Leibnitz served three consecutive rulers of the House of Brunswick as historian, political adviser, and most consequentially, as librarian of the Ducal library, all professions which fall under the auspices of the empirical wise man. Hence he will be discussing one of the empirical wise man's favorite topics, how these two substances (the Descartes version of the mind and body)—or two experiences (the Spinoza version of the mind and body)—could possibly interact. His answer? It's what they have in common that connects them—they interact over time. In other words, it's our sense of time which joins our experiences of the mind and body. Realize this is just another way to describe what happens in stories. Literally, a story tells how things do and do not interact over time.

Who then will represent the rationalist wise man? Professor Johann Friedrich Herbart, Immanuel Kant's successor as chair of philosophy at Königsberg when Kant died. In part, he's drawn this assignment because he attempted to create an algebra which describes human nature. Talk about rational. But the main reason is that his work allows us to combine the prior three viewpoints. Thus the least known man, Herbart, holds the key to this mystery, in that he'll be doing what the rationalist wise man loves to do best—he'll give us the overarching view.

Know that each of these men could easily represent all four wise men. They're all geniuses in their own right, as you're about to see. Please treat this discussion, then, as a sort of grand debate wherein there are four teams and where each philosopher has been somewhat randomly assigned a position to defend, *somewhat* being the operative word.

Above all, the thing to watch for will be this. While, on the surface, these four views will seem completely incompatible, in reality, all four are equally true. Thus what makes this discussion particularly salient is that it is a clear and distinct example of how, by combining the wisdom of the four wise men, you can arrive at a personal truth. In effect, you're going to see for yourself how powerful this truth-finding method can be, given you can open your mind and body to the wisdom in all four wise men's viewpoints, as well as to the wisdom in you.

Before We Start, a Quick Review of the Playbill

By the way, if you're put off by the thought of yet more head-deadening philosophy, don't worry. The focus of most of this chapter will be on stories, not theory. At the same time, because stories are what give theories their meaning, it's important that you do your best to picture these stories. Only then will you be able to grasp the secrets being revealed here.

Okay. So before I start throwing stuff at the fan, let's review the playbill. To begin with, I'm going to set the stage by telling you two stories from my practice as a therapist—the stories of Audrey and Lori, the two women who got me thinking about where we get our sense of time. Next we'll briefly look at the work of Dr. Michael D. Gershon, a neurobiologist whose work centers on that we have two physiological brains. His work addresses the physical aspects of the mind body mystery and explains where we get our sense of time from—we get it from sensing temporal differences between our two physiological brains.

Next we'll address the psychological aspects of the mind body mystery, beginning with our four philosophers, each of whom will offer an explanation as to why we sense the mind and body separately. And how they could interact. First up will be René Descartes, who will present the materialist wise man's point of view—that it comes from a material dualism. Baruch de Spinoza will then defend the spiritual wise man's position—that it comes from a spiritual unity. Gottfried Wilhelm von Leibnitz will then argue for the empirical wise man's position—that it comes from how things interact over time. Then Professor Johann Friedrich Herbart will close with the rationalist wise man's position—that the truth must be an overarching view which combines all these opinions.

Finally, I'm going to show you how you can test this two brains thing yourself, beginning with exploring the differences between "science teacher's time" and the two kinds of "personal time." Which brain do you favor anyway, your mind's brain or your body's? Can you guess at this point? I promise, by the end of this chapter, you'll have a clear and distinct answer, so clear in fact that I suspect you'll never feel or think about time the same way again.

So now, are you ready for me to turn on the fan? Then climb up into the theoria and fasten your seat belt. Mind body bloodbath, here we come.

Audrey's Story—A Mind Before Body Person

We're going to start with Audrey's story. Audrey is one of the two women I mentioned a moment ago who raised questions in me about where we get our sense of time. She's also a world famous classical musician whose fans, and students, fawn over her. Deservedly. Can you imagine my surprise then when she asked me for help with a musical problem? To put it mildly, I was taken aback. The problem? She had played an opera wherein a guest conductor had paced the orchestra noticeably faster than usual. So much so, in fact, that she told me she had struggled to keep up. Being as I sang on records as a kid and had been humiliated on more than one occasion for being out of time, I felt an immediate connection to her. And yes. I'm well aware I am not in her league. Not even remotely. Still, compassion is rooted in similarity, not in ratings. Thus when she told me this, my heart went out to her.

To be honest, I also felt a bit awkward doing what I did next—I asked her to sing part of the melody while tapping her leg. The result? I was stunned. She could not do it and stay in time. Imagine my disbelief. How could a world class musician, at the top of her game for decades, be having this kind of trouble? It was literally beyond my ability to comprehend. So much so that I asked her to try doing this several more times, all with the same outcome. She couldn't get her voice and her hand in sync.

Then it hit me. I realized that Audrey's problem had nothing to do with her level of skill. It stemmed from that we have two different senses of time, not just one. In Audrey's case, it was her mind's sense of time that was supervising her singing, and her body's sense of time that was conducting her tapping hand. Moreover, the harder she tried to mentally urge her body and mind into sync, the more her hand lagged behind her voice, just as it had with that conductor's hand.

How about you? Have you ever witnessed this kind of thing—someone whose mind races ahead of their mouth? To be honest, I cannot count the number of times I've seen people do this. Or done this myself. Yet until that moment, it had never occurred to me to frame this as a mind body problem—as that the mind and body were out of sync. Duh. I now realize this was what Yogi Berra was referring to when he said *you can't think and bat*. Or think and do any body oriented activity. Think and dance. Think and sing. Think and play a musical instrument. Think and play a sport.

Please realize, I'm not saying doing these things requires no intelligence. The mind is often the prelude to doing these things well. But when it comes time to actually do these things, the time to think is over. Do them without thinking and you'll more likely do them well.

At this point, I'd suggest you take a moment to let what I've just introduced sink in. To begin with, try to set aside what I'm claiming these observations mean and just answer this. Have you seen this happen? Have you seen someone whose mind is racing ahead of their body? Hell, have you had this happen to you? I have. More times than I care to remember. I sucked at playing baseball and at all sports in fact. I tried, briefly, to learn to play guitar and sucked at that too. And learning to play piano, well, I felt like I had four hands. And in a way, I did—the two on the ends of my arms, and the two in my head.

Are you getting what I'm saying here? We get our personal sense of time—not the science teacher's time, mind you, but rather our personal sense of time—from two places. One. We get it from the sense of time we keep in our mind. Two. We get it from the sense of time we keep in our body. In Audrey's case, the clock in her mind was running faster than the clock in her body, so much so that the more she tried to mentally control her hand, the faster she sang and the more her hand lagged behind, this from a world class musician, no less.

Let me say this again. What I saw that day, for the first time ever, was that we have two ways to keep time. Moreover, the proficiency of everything we do rests on how well these two clocks sync up. More important, this explains how we can have the sense that the mind and body are separate. As far as time is concerned, they are separate. And because time, besides being a psychological reality, is also a physical reality, we literally have a separate mind and body.

Have I just annoyed the crap out of you by repeating this idea so many times? Then maybe it's time I make my point. This idea—that we have two senses of time, is the most important idea in this book. Period. That I'm basing this idea on both a physical reality (having two physical brains) and a psychological reality (having two senses of time) only underscores the validity of this idea further. Moreover, the idea that the mind and body compete for dominance with regard to time explains a whole lot about who we are, including not only how we can experience the mind and body as two separate kinds of personal consciousness, but also why having them sync up feels so good it's like dying and going to heaven. It is heaven to be playing music and feel like you're in the groove, or to play a sport and feel like you're in the zone, or to meditate and feel like you're one with all things, or to be a scientist and finally get the aha. These things occur only when the mind and body are in sync. And the battle for mind body dominance is why they so rarely do.

What does all this mean? In Audrey's case, it means that her mind was dominating over her body. Her rational and spiritual truths were overriding her empirical and material truths. However, like all truths, to see what this means, we must now look at what it feels like to have the exact opposite experience—the body dominating over the mind. That this was supplied to me in spades just two days later only reminds me yet again that all truth lies on continuums of polar opposites. To wit, what I needed to see to complete this picture was that the opposite condition is also possible—that the body can race ahead of the mind. This is what Lori supplied. But not before she pointed out that I was just like Audrey.

Lori's Story—A Body Before Mind Person

Lori is a woman whom I've known for years. She's also someone whom I openly admit to having fatherly feelings for, and she's shared similar thoughts with me. To wit, Lori once told me, many years ago, that she wished I was her father. Being as I've never had good relationships with my own children, you can imagine how this felt. To both of us.

What you can't imagine though is how I feel about her mind. Lori is one of the smartest people I know, albeit, whenever I tell her this, she silently and respectfully blows me off. You see, Lori's got one of the worst cases of ADHD I've ever seen, including that she has trouble recalling her accomplishments five minutes later. The result? Lori's brilliant mind is constantly fighting to emerge from her dominant body. Moreover, whenever you ask her a question, her mind goes blank and her body gets more active, whereas whenever you give her a compliment, she thinks you're just patronizing or ridiculing her. To Lori, most ideas are surreal and can't be trusted, whereas whatever her body tells her she believes.

Admittedly, helping Lori has been part of what's been motivating me to solve the ADHD mystery. That several of my closest friends also have it has only deepened my desire. How meaningful, then, that Lori is the one who opened the door for me on what ADHD is, just by making a single, spontaneous, off-the-cuff remark about something she saw me doing. At the time, I was explaining something to her and was simultaneously trying to diagram it for her on a pad. Wherein, she remarked, totally out of the blue and in a somewhat surprised manner, that my hand couldn't keep up with my words.

My hand couldn't keep up with my words. Does this at all sound like what I've just told you about Audrey—that her hand couldn't keep up with her mouth? Okay, I thought. So our minds run faster than our bodies. Moreover, when I considered how this could be explained by simple physics—that non physical thoughts move faster than physical bodies—it made sense. However, when I asked Lori if she too was like this, she told me she was just the opposite—that her hand leads her mouth. Sure enough, when we tried it, she drew first, then spoke. Her body ran ahead of her mind.

I knew at this point that what I had seen in these two women couldn't be explained away by mere physics. If this was the case, all people would be the same, varying only in degree. That I saw in Lori the exact opposite response from Audrey was almost proof enough for the two brains theory. But when I framed Lori's ADHD as a mind body problem, as in you can't bat and think, I was hooked. And yes, we've a ways to go before I expect you to see why I'm so sure about this. Much of chapter twelve in Book III will address this topic. For now, all I ask is this. Try to see what I've been telling you here as the process I went through as I searched for a solution to the mind body mystery.

This brings us to the next installment, the physiological source for our two senses of time, our two physiological brains.

Dr. Gershon and the Second Brain

Of course, the question in my mind at this point was, where the heck are these two women getting their sense of time from—the physiological source? At which point, I remembered reading a book by a Dr. Michael D. Gershon, a neurobiologist whose work centers around proving that we have two brains. Not two rational brains, mind you. The one in our head is quite enough, thank you very much. Rather, he says we have a second, fully independent "lower" brain sandwiched in the collective lining of the esophagus, stomach, intestines, and colon diaphragm.

Realize what I'm saying here. Dr. Gershon says we literally have two physically separate brains. A brain in the head. And a brain in the bowel. Please know that when he writes this, he is not merely referring to this second brain metaphorically, or behaviorally. Nor is he positing a medically unsupported, neurological absurdity. Rather, he is referring to what medical doctors call, *the enteric nervous system*, a complex system of nerves and nerve centers in and around the gut which literally function as a separate and distinct "brain." His words, not mine.

What makes him say this so emphatically? If you'll forgive my lay retelling, I'm going to attempt to break down what he says into five, bite sized chunks, while adding in a chunk of my own. Stand back from the fan, please.

Proof #1—The Number of Cells Present

There are more that one hundred million nerve cells in the enteric nervous system, more than in the entire spine, and more than in the entire remainder of the peripheral nervous system. Is this number much smaller than the number of cells in the cranial brain? Substantially. The brain in the head has something like a thousand times as many cells. Realize though that this is like saying your computer has two megs of RAM as opposed to two gigs. There are computers which run on two megs of RAM. More slowly, of course. But they run. And one hundred million nerve cells is still a heck of a lot of cells. In fact, many animals have fully functioning brains with far fewer neurons.

Proof #2—The Kinds of Cells Present

If we compare levels of structural complexity present in the designs of these two brains, it's no contest. The brain in the head wins hands down. Even so, when it comes to the kinds of nerve cells present, they're pretty much the same. In fact, the brain in the gut contains every class of neurotransmitter the brain in the head contains. This includes not only major neurotransmitters like serotonin, dopamine, glutamate, norephinephrine and nitric oxide, but also two dozen neuropeptides (small brain proteins), endorphins (a chemical relative to opiates), benzodiazepines (the main ingredient in valium and xanax), and the major cells of the immune system. Quite a diversity of cells, don't you think?

Are these cells anywhere else in the body?

Not in these large numbers.

Proof #3—The Amount of Serotonin Present

Neurotransmitters are like old fashioned bicycle messengers, only they carry messages between nerves. Serotonin is one of the main neurotransmitters, and the messages it carries are largely about moods. This is why most current antidepressant medications are SSRIs—selective serotonin reuptake inhibitors. Depression is a condition wherein we have too few mood-messages being delivered, and SSRIs fool the body into thinking there is more serotonin present than there actually is by making these deliveries take longer.

The thing is, when we talk about where these medications work, we assume they work in the head. But it's a proven fact that 80-95% of the serotonin in the body is made, and exists, not in the head, but in the gut. So where is the Prozac working? You tell me. And what is the gut's role in depression and in other psychological problems?

Interestingly enough, in the opening of his book, Dr. Gershon hints at this possibility when he says, *Since the enteric nervous system can function on its own, it must be considered possible that the brain in the bowel may also have its own psychoneuroses.* Moreover, while neither of us are suggesting that the brain in the gut is the main source of psychological problems, it surely must play a significant role. How could it not? The overwhelming majority of mood-message deliveries occur in the gut.

Proof #4—The Scope of What Serotonin Affects

What else besides mood does serotonin affect? Start with this. Doctors tell us that serotonin's effects are normally inhibitory. In other words, serotonin diminishes things. For instance, the absence of serotonin has been correlated with an increase of aggressive behavior, so it's presence is assumed to inhibit aggression. There is also a strong correlation between serotonin levels and appetite as in, too little and we overeat, and too much and we undereat. Serotonin also affects our sleep and wake cycles (circadian rhythm) as in, too little and we sleep more, and too much and we can't sleep. And it is also correlated to being irritable, to being impulsive, and is said to affect our sexual desire, body temperature, metabolism, and pain perception.

Am I saying that changes in serotonin levels, in and of themselves, cause, impair, or cure any of this? Not at all. Thus, by *correlated to*, I mean *coexists with*, not *causes*. Still, serotonin is the chemical messenger which communicates, or fails to communicate, the instructions for all these things. Hence, again, I'm simply saying it is a major player in these parts of our lives.

Proof #5—How All This Connects to Our Sense of Time

Did you notice how many things serotonin affects? Anger, aggression, irritability, impulsivity, body temperature, and sleep cycles, as well as sexuality, appetite, pain regulation, and metabolism. Serotonin even stimulates vomiting. Now take a minute to consider what all these things have in common. Anger, aggression, impulsivity, irritability, body temperature, pain regulation, sleep cycles, appetite, sexuality, metabolism, and vomiting. Have you ever experienced of any of these things and had a sense of *time-over-time*? In other words, have you ever experienced these things and done anything other than focus on what was happening right there in the moment? I haven't. Nor has anyone I know. And yes, I know of many women who think about their laundry or plan meals while having sex. But in reality, you can't have sex without being there. So these ladies are not having sex. They are thinking about their laundry and planning meals.

The point is, the commonality in all these serotonin-related things is that they're all *one-moment-at-a-time* events. When you're in them, you're focused only on what's happening in the present moment. And when you're not, then you're not doing them. They're being done to you.

Are you beginning to see why the brain in the gut would sense time as one-moment-at-a-time? And how our two physiological brains, and the two ways we can sense time, are tied to the two experiences we call mind and body?

Proof #6—Functional Independence

The icing on the two brains cake, of course, is that the brain in the gut is completely capable of functioning without input from the brain in the head. What I'm saying is, if you sever the nerves which connect the brain or spinal cord to any limb or organ *other than the gut*, this limb or organ will no longer function. This includes the heart, the lungs, the liver, the bladder, the kidneys, the skeletal muscles, the pancreas, the adrenals, and so on. In the case of the gut, however, if you do this, it will still function fine. Moreover, this is true even to the point wherein you can surgically remove parts of the gut from the body, and if you keep them alive, they will still continue to function. Surprising? Yes. But controversial? Not at all. This is a known biological fact. And lest you think I'm misinterpreting Dr. Gershon, allow me to quote the good doctor in his own words. He says, the gut is *the only organ that contains an intrinsic nervous system that is able to mediate reflexes in the complete absence of input from the brain or spinal cord.*

One more point. The number of nerve fibers which connect these two brains is notably small. Only one to two thousand nerve fibers connect

them. Compare this to the number of nerve fibers which connect the eyes
to the brain in the head—over one million.

Functional independence. Do you get the implications of this? The gut
is different from the rest of the body in that, even in the complete absence
of input from the brain and spinal cord, it still continues to function. That
this happens to parts of it even if you surgically remove them from the
body is astounding. Why? Because for this to happen, the gut must still
be getting instructions. Not from the brain in the head or from the spine,
mind you, but rather from the enteric nervous system itself.

This in part is why Dr. Gershon calls the gut, the "second brain."
Granted, he in no way means this brain can do calculus or teach chemistry.
Clearly, we are talking here only about lower bodily functions. However, for
any function to occur, it must include instructions. And giving instructions
which vary in ways which are far more complex than simple to-do lists is
one of the two things which make something a brain, the other being the
ability to direct the timing of these instructions—in other words, having
a sense of time.

Oddly, Dr. Gershon never mentions this second item, perhaps because
having a sense of time is seen more as existing within the domain of
psychologists and so, is not his area. Yet, in order for a brain to issue
instructions and direct activities, it must have a sense of when and when
not to do these things. Moreover, this brain must either get its sense of
time from elsewhere or have its own intrinsic sense of time—its own
master clock. And in the case of the brain in the gut, clearly, it contains
its own master clock.

What makes this so important? Because if indeed we do respond
separately to what we feel in our gut, then knowing this separateness exists
physiologically as well as psychologically adds yet one more pointer in
the direction of mind body dualism and Descartes. And yes, Dr. Gershon
himself wisely avoids this topic completely, something I respect him for
doing. He has, in fact, on numerous occasions refused to acknowledge, or
deny, that this second brain is responsible for our "gut reactions." Given
how often doctors have been known to crucify their peers for even alluding
to such things publicly, I find this a sane choice on his part. After all, his
area of expertise is the body, not the mind. Considering all you've just
heard though, do you have any doubt that we have two physical brains?
And yes, structurally, these two brains are extremely different, so much
so in fact that some neurobiologists refuse to accept the existence of

the brain in the gut simply because it does not compare structurally to the brain in the head. This is akin to saying an abacus is not a computer simply because it does not have a hard drive and can't burn DVDs. Even so, [1] because the brain in the gut is capable of giving instructions which fractally vary even with no input whatsoever from the brain in the head, and [2] because these instructions include their own method of sensing time—*one-moment-at-a-time,* as opposed to the brain in the head's way of sensing time—as *time-over-time,* it's clear, we have two physical brains.

Now let's move away from the physical aspects of the mind body mystery and onto the psychological aspects. Four wise men, get on your mark. Witnesses, move back from the fan.

Descartes' Interaction Puzzle—His Two Kinds of Matter

René Descartes made four assumptions about the mind body connection. One. He said that the experiences of the mind and the experiences of the body are different. Two. He said that what makes these experiences different is that they originate in two entirely different substances, one with and one without extension. Three. He said these two different substances interact with each other. Mind affecting body. And body affecting mind. And four. He said there is a literal mechanism through which these two separate but interactive substances connect.

The problem, of course, centers mainly on how two completely different substances, one which takes up space and one which doesn't, could ever interact. This is like saying that an immaterial being, a ghost for instance, can interact with a material being like us. This idea prompted British philosopher, Gilbert Ryle, to write a book mocking Descartes' dualism, calling it "the dogma of the ghost in the machine" (*The Concept of Mind*, Gilbert Ryle, The University of Chicago Press, Chicago, 1949). Here, Ryle claims that unless you can prove how the mind and body interact, it's nonsense to say they do.

Despite Ryle's book being both dated and flawed, he makes a valid point. For Descartes to be right about the mind and body being two substances, we need to understand how they can coexist and interact. At the same time, to require, as Ryle does, that this proof be based on the kinds of measurements materialists demand, i.e. facts, ignores Descartes' definitions and is patently absurd. Facts by definition only measure physical things, things which take up space. But the mind by definition is not physical and therefore, does not take up space. How then can our inability to physically measure the mind be proof it does not exist?

Where does this leave us then? Let's start at the beginning with Descartes' opening assumption—that we experience life in two basic ways—first, as mental experiences; as the experiences of a mind, and second, as physical experiences; as the experiences of a body. So do we experience life in these two ways? Duh. Do bowels emit foul odors. Of course, we do. In fact, while Ryle himself takes every opportunity to ridicule dualism, he also does quite a good job describing what these two kinds of experiences feel like.

The Point? Regardless of whether we do or do not accept the rest of Descartes' ideas, the fact is, we certainly do experience life from the viewpoint of a living, biological dualism—as a mind and a body. No one argues about this. What we argue about is whether this experience is based on an illusion or a measurable, material reality. So which is it? Fortunately, the answer is easier to see than most people realize. All we need do is review what we said in the last chapter about the difference between *substances without extension*—Descartes' way of defining what the mind is made of—and the way physicists define *energy*. Not the incorporeal kinds of energy, mind you, the kinds ghost hunters and psychics claim exist. Rather, we are talking about the kinds of observable energies absorbed, utilized, and emitted by the human body.

This then is the first thing to realize about Descartes' two substances. When Descartes says the mind derives from a substance without extension, in today's language, he's saying that the mind is made of energy. Do materialists accept energy as a material reality? Duh! Do we need to talk about bears' bathroom habits again? Of course, they do. So why don't they see the mind as energy? It's simple—because they reify the concept of energy. And for those for whom this word is unfamiliar (and for those who did not read my comments on this word in the last chapter's notes written in the margin), allow me to explain.

To *reify* means to regard or treat an abstraction as if it has a concrete or material existence. So when I say we "reify the concept of energy," I'm saying we treat energy, which is just a concept, as if it's a literal, physical thing. It's not. Energy is just a word we use to describe changes which occur in matter. And if you don't believe me, look it up. In particular, note how this word is defined in physics. To a physicist, energy is the capacity of a physical system to do work.

So is "the capacity to do work" a measurable substance *with* extension? In other words, does "the capacity to do work" occupy space? For most people, trying to make sense of these two sentences will result in their brains farting. Why? Because asking these two questions is like asking if any words which denote action, the words our high school English teachers called *verbs*, take up space.

For example, consider what's happening in the sentence, *I watched in horror as the autumn wind blew my lazy neighbor's brown crinkled leaves into my recently manicured azalia bushes.* The *leaves* take up space. So does the *wind*. But does what happened to those leaves—*blew*, take up space? Yes, *blowing* occurs within space. But is *blowing* a measurable substance with extension—a physical thing? Or is *blowing* a verb, meaning, something which describes how physical things like leaves change?

Admittedly the idea of *reifying* concepts can be hard to understand. We do it so often, we rarely if ever notice. For instance, when we say we have more "energy," what we actually have more of is not anything physical. Rather, we have more ability to change some sort of matter. Thus whether it's the wind blowing leaves into your azalia bushes, or you blasting your lazy neighbor for allowing this to happen—either way, saying we have the energy to do these things says only that we have the capacity to do these things, and not that we possess anything physical.

Not surprisingly, Thomas Young, the originator of the term *energy*, never used this word to refer to something physical. Rather, he too defined it as "the ability to do work." In fact, the Greek word he drew on, *energeia*, means "activity" or "operation." So when modern physicists define energy—not as a kind of matter, but rather as something which has the power to effect or change matter—this is why. As well as why we never actually see energy. We see only the effect it has on matter, including when we use test equipment such as volt-ohm meters and light meters. In reality, these meters measure only the effect an energy has on some kind of matter.

What about Einstein's famous formula wherein he equates energy to matter? Here again, we see how a wise man's words can confuse the issue. Equating something to something else does not mean they're literally the same. It means only that in some significant way, they are similar enough to be called equivalents, similar to how Italians equate a fart in the breeze to things which are extremely transient.

So is energy itself measurable? In reality, no. Not directly, anyway. Even so, no modern materialist would deny that this substance *without* extension, i.e. energy, affects and interacts with substances *with* extension, i.e. matter. By never questioning the actual meaning of the term *energy* though, they preserve their right to ridicule the other wise men's beliefs. Including that they feel entitled to call Descartes' belief in substances without extension, *the dogma of the ghost in the machine.*

Are you getting this? The modern physicist's *concept of energy* is literally the same as Descartes' *substance without extension*. Which is why, when materialists claim to be able to measure energy, they never actually measure energy. They measure only the effect this energy has on matter. In truth, then, our world is filled with substances without extension which affect substances with extension and vice versa. Yet even when faced with direct proof for this, such as when electrical energy affects a light bulb (when it lights the light bulb) and vice versa (when the lit filament causes electrical resistance), materialists somehow refuse to see this as proof that Descartes' two substances, one with and one without extension, can affect each other.

Not feeling comfortable with how I am equating the mind with energy? Then consider how materialist neuro researchers claim to be able to measure the mind. They measure the energies they've come to associate with the functioning of the brain. Of course, this then raises the obvious question. How do we know, with certainty, whether these electro-chemical interactions equate to what we call the mind? The answer. We don't. Moreover, despite claims by some researchers that their tests reveal the inner workings of the brain, it will likely be a long time, if ever, before we can intelligently correlate what we see in fMRIs, CAT and PET scans, SPECT, and electrophysiological testing such as electroencephalography (EEG) or magnetoencephalography (MEG), to the actual workings of the mind.

What makes me say this? If you understand the temporal limitations of these tests, you realize how far these researchers must stretch the data to make their interpretations. Thoughts happen instantaneously. These machines take a much longer time to register and record their data. In addition, do you realize how bold it is to claim to be able to correlate this data to the psychologically soft data of subjective reporting and personal interactions? Holy shit. In truth, these scientists are claiming to be able to read minds. Doesn't sound too scientific to me. Talk about ghosts in machines.

Fortunately, none of this matters. Nor do we need to wait for this dilemma to be resolved. You see, there is an easy, direct, logically sound way to materially demonstrate the mind body difference. One which satisfies even the materialist wise man. How? All I'm going to say at this point is this. There is a test which proves there is a separate mind and body, and this test involves manipulating the very thing which limits the value of the neuro researcher's tests—time. All I ask you to allow for at this point are two things. One. That we have two very different ways to experience life, as a being with a mind and as a being with a body. And two. That the modern physicist's *concept of energy* is literally the same as Descartes' *substance without extension*. Can you live with this? Do these things feel true to you? If so, then we're ready to move on to our second philosopher, Baruch de Spinoza.

Spinoza's Solution—All Matter Derives From One Source

René Descartes was thirty six years old when Spinoza was born. So when Descartes published his *Discourse on Method*, Spinoza was five. However, being as the *Discourse* was the seventeenth century equivalent of a bestseller, Spinoza was most certainly exposed to it early in life. Originally, he was said to have agreed with Descartes, that body and mind are two separate substances. Indeed, he appears to have been greatly affected by Descartes' ideas, so much so in fact that in 1663, he even published a geometric "clarification" of Descartes' ideas, Parts I and II of *Descartes' Principles of Philosophy*. Not long after this, however, he began work on what would eventually become his best known work, his *Ethics*, which was completed somewhere around 1676 and published only after his death in 1677. In it, Spinoza clearly embraces the existence of dualism, but only as two attributes of one and the same thing—*Deus sive natura* (God or nature).

Know that when Spinoza refers to "God or nature," he uses these two words interchangeably. To him, they were merely two names for the same universal, underlying substance. Here Spinoza defines this substance not as "matter" but rather as "that which stands beneath"—"that whose concept doesn't have to be formed out of the concept of something else." He then goes on to say that while this substance has an infinite number of attributes, human beings are able to perceive only two—thought and extension—and that it is from these two attributes that we get our experiences of mind and body.

So is he right? Are all things, including the mind and body, manifestations of one and the same substance? According to the spiritual wise man, yes. This is the only possible truth. At the same time, Spinoza admits we can never directly know this universal substance, only its two knowable attributes. Hence our belief that the mind and body are two separate and distinct substances.

Are you following this? According to Descartes, we experience life as a body and as a mind. Moreover, because these two experiences differ greatly, we conclude the world is made of two different substances, one of which takes up space and one which doesn't. Spinoza agrees but says that, in reality, all experience derives from the same nameless stuff. And while this universal stuff has an infinite number of attributes, we can know only two—thought and extension. The rest remain unknowable.

So who is right? Descartes and the materialist wise man who say that mind and body are two opposite and distinctly different substances? Or Spinoza and the spiritual wise man who say that mind and body are two attributes of the one universal substance? Can we even know? And why all the fuss over these two views anyway?

Obviously we have these two experiences. If we didn't, none of this would matter to us. The problem has been how to explain these two experiences. Where do they come from? Descartes says they come from the two distinctly different but interactive substances from which we are made, one of which takes up space, and one of which does not.

But if this is so and these two substances interact, why can't we physically measure this interaction?

Here Spinoza offers us a sensible answer—he uses monism to answer this question. He says the mind and body appear to interact because in reality, they differ only in appearance. Beneath this appearance, however, they are actually one and the same substance, making the apparent interactions two properties of the same event.

The problem with this answer of course is that this is a metaphysical answer, and metaphysical answers rarely if ever satisfy those seeking observable answers. However, if we visually combine Spinoza's unseen, underlying *continuum-of-substance* (monism) with Descartes' *two substances* (dualism), we get an interesting result. We get an observable composite which begins to reveal how this connection could exist. In theory, anyway.

Now take a moment to consider how we've arrived at this composite. We've used a method I've referred to several times before. We've taken a pair of opposites and made them the end points of a single continuum, and in doing this, we've treated these two explanations as if they are the first two of the five aspects from the last chapter—the two sides (duality) and one coin (unity) views.

Interestingly enough, while doing research on this section, I noticed Spinoza uses this same coin analogy in his *Ethics*. Having come to it independently in the last chapter, I have to admit, this felt good. As for where these two explanations leave us, admittedly, they give us only a starting point—a possible material solution to the interaction question. We've still got to explain what prevents us from seeing Spinoza's continuum, as well as how this duality connects psychologically. Before moving on to address these two questions, however, we'll first need to take a deeper look at how the ideas of our first two philosophers connect visually.

Compositing All Four Viewpoints in One Diagram

If you now look at the diagram on the next page, the one I've titled, *How The Mind And Body Connect (as seen through the eyes of the four philosophers)*, you'll find I've combined the viewpoints of all four philosophers into a single diagram. Here, I've numbered these viewpoints, one through four—beginning with Descartes and his *two substances*; mind *and* body, which I've designated as number one—followed by Spinoza's *continuum-of-substance*; mind *to* body, which I've designated as number two.

Now take a closer look at this drawing. Can you see how Descartes' *two substances* version of the mind and body is represented by what appear to be two waves of experience, separate above the midline and flowing into each other below this line? Can you also see how Spinoza's *two attributes* version of the mind and body—the horizontal continuum below these two waves—describes the flow from mind to body as a gradual change within a single continuum of substance?

The main thing to notice, of course, is how this combined view neither attempts to prove nor deny either explanation. Rather, in this drawing, neither way of thinking is wrong, and both add something to what we know. Can you see how the drawing accomplishes this? Because all four explanations intersect and overlap, your sense of what is true changes based on where you look, sort of like you are experiencing the eyes of a theoretical Mona Lisa. Move your focus and your sense of what is true moves too.

Know that these kinds of changes happen within all personal truths. Which is why we call this, changing our viewpoint. This leaves us with but one way to arrive at a personal truth. We must take in the entire drawing in the same way in which we take in a work of art, not in pieces, but rather as a whole experience. Only then can you hope to arrive at a personal appreciation of what you see, the beauty in what's in front of you.

Easier said than done, you say? You're right. But you can learn. Indeed, were you to take an art appreciation course, you'd likely gain a lot of the skills necessary to find truth. This same idea may even have been what prompted Keats to write, "Beauty is truth, truth beauty, that is all ye know on earth, and all ye need to know" (*Ode to A Grecian Urn*, from *The Poetical Works of John Keats*, John Keats, Macmillan, London, 1884). Amazing how the fractal for truth repeats itself in so many seemingly dissimilar areas of life.

How the Mind and Body Connect
(as seen through the eyes of the four philosophers)
(© 2007 Steven Paglierani The Center for Emergence)

The Mind and Body as Two Interactive Experiences
René Descartes (1596 - 1650)
Descartes hypothesized that the mind and body were
two different substances, both of which interacted with the
other. Thus Descartes's contribution is that we experience the
mind and body as two separate but interactive experiences.

The Mind and Body as Connected by Time
Freidrich Wilhelm Leibniz (1646 - 1716)
Leibniz hypothesized that the mind and body were two different
substances, both of which resembled watches set by God at birth so as
to be running in perfect sync. Thus Leibniz's contribution is the idea
that what connects the mind and body is our two experiences of time.

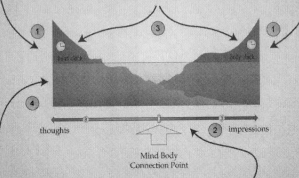

thoughts   Mind Body Connection Point   impressions

The Mind and Body as One Continuum
(Baruch) Benedictus de Spinoza (1632 - 1677)
Spinoza hypothesized that the mind and body were two aspects of the
same thing and that this thing was God. Thus Spinoza's contribution is
that the mind and body are in fact two ends of the same continuum.

The Mind and Body as Having a Threshold of Perception
Johann Freidrich Herbart (1776 - 1841)
Herbart hypothesized that we experienced the mind and body only
when the intensity of these experiences crossed above a threshold of
consciousness. Thus Herbart's contribution is the idea that it is the
intensity of our experiences of the mind and body which allows us
to know they exist, moreover that there are mind body experiences
which fall below this threshold of perception.

So what do you think? Can you see how accurately our first two philosophers' views describe the differences between how we experience the material world and how we experience the spiritual world? And if you don't believe in a spiritual world? Then try to see this second view as the underlying, invisible world of the physicist's energy, the stuff we can never directly see or measure except as an effect on matter.

Remember too that we're not looking here for the ultimate truth about the mind and body, as in what feels true to all people. We're trying to find personal truth, as in what feels true to you. Moreover, as we've defined it, a personal truth is never as insignificant as a personal opinion. Rather, it's what emerges in you when you and all four wise men agree on something. This said, isn't it amazing how seeing the truth in two such dissimilar explanations—Descartes' and Spinoza's—so depends on being able to visually combine their two viewpoints into a single picture?

Here then is one of the more important things to see about the truth finding method I'm describing in this series of books. Seeing all four viewpoints does not mean merely knowing they exist. Nor does it mean getting a good feel for them. Rather, it means literally integrating all four wise men's views into a single, clear and distinct picture. No clear and distinct picture. No personal truth. And yes, by saying we must have a "picture," this can appear to challenge the conventional wisdom which says we each have different learning styles—kinesthetic, visual, tactile, etc. However, what it's really saying is that our learning style must lead to a picture which we can experience kinesthetically, visually, tactilely, and so on.

Are you getting this? To arrive at a personal truth, you must visually integrate the wisdom of all four wise men into a single picture. In addition, you must do this in a way in which nothing is dismissed, denied, belittled, or left out. And yes, learning to create these kinds of pictures can involve some brain-twisting work, including that you must have an extremely open mind. However, since we're nowhere near the point where you should be trying to do this, you need not worry if this drawing still evokes more discomfort than a class in hieroglyphics.

At the same time, the more you understand this drawing, the closer you'll be to creating your own drawings. And to finding your personal truth. With this in mind, it might even be worth your while to try your hand at redrawing this picture, one philosopher at a time, of course, and only after I've introduced the remaining two wise men. Will this guarantee you'll understand this drawing? Not really. However, the more familiar you become with these drawings, the easier it will be to make your own.

How will you know you've grasped what is in this drawing?

You'll feel pleasantly surprised by what you see. For instance, you may be surprised by how easily this simple diagram resolves the disparate viewpoints of four such dissimilar philosophers. Imagine being able to resolve all such disagreements—in effect, being able to see the whole picture even with someone with whom you strongly disagree? You can, if you learn how to make these drawings, then look for pleasant surprises.

Does this sound overly simple, or too optimistic? If so, then perhaps it would help you to remember which wise man is saying this—the rationalist wise man. This makes my statement true only in theory. Thus it's open to all sorts of failures in the real world.

Even so, there's no denying that in a very tangible way, this simple drawing accomplishes something most people can't do. In effect, two opposing viewpoints are being treated as equally true. In other words, below the midline, we have the idea that all things are attributes of the one wondrous all, making us all equally beautiful and right in God's eyes. This thoroughly mirrors Spinoza's philosophy and the spiritual wise man's teachings. At the same time, above the midline, we've got the idea that the mind and body are two different and distinctly opposite substances. Here, we find Descartes' philosophy and the materialist wise man's position.

Can you see how different this is from how people normally resolve disputes? Most folks either abstain from arguing, argue and fight that their viewpoint is right, argue that there can logically be only one right viewpoint, or argue that one viewpoint is mainly right with a little bit of the other views thrown in for good measure.

For instance, in the case of the mind body mystery, this is how people have been trying to solve this mystery for centuries now. Yet all along, there's been a way to resolve these opposing arguments.

Admittedly, this method—compositing opposing viewpoints into a single visual truth—is counterintuitive. But it works nonetheless.

So now, let me ask you. Is it beginning to dawn on you how combining the four wise men's viewpoints might lead to a personal truth? Granted, we've a ways to go before you'll be able to do this on your own. I haven't even introduced you to the other two philosophers yet, let alone to the six step method which enables you to create these drawings. This said, if you've been open minded, even at this point you should be feeling hints of what is to come. Speaking of which, you might be interested to know that Spinoza concluded that feelings stem from *inadequate understanding*. Having previously defined feelings as what emerges from us when we experience things which are beyond words, this is interesting, is it not?

Now let's move on to our next philosopher, the man who will present the empirical wise man's point of view. Who knows, maybe we'll find some parallels to our present endeavor in his philosophy as well.

Leibnitz's Solution—The Two Kinds of Matter Exist in Sync

Gottfried Leibnitz was born in 1646, fourteen years after Spinoza and right before Descartes died. Thus he wasn't alive in 1637 when Descartes published his *Discourse on Method*. Like Spinoza though, he was profoundly affected by Descartes' ideas. As well as by Spinoza's, whose ideas he harshly rebuked in an unfinished book published years after his death as *Refutation of Spinoza*. To his credit, Leibnitz appears to never have intended to publish this book. In effect, it's merely a collection of notes he wrote to himself in the margins of Spinoza's *Ethics*. At the same time, these notes offer us some insight into the nature of the man. Leibnitz was a profoundly gentle, well mannered, but intensely analytic soul. To wit, most of these notes point out logical contradictions in Spinoza's ideas.

I mention this because in a way it makes Leibnitz's solution to the mind body interaction mystery seem rather odd. In it, he combines logic and metaphysics into a story about God. His solution? Leibnitz says the mind and body each have their own sense of time, their own clock so to speak. He then goes on to say that, at birth, God sets these two clocks in perfect sync, and that forever more, they remain in sync throughout a person's lifetime.

To Leibnitz then, whenever the mind seems to be affecting the body—or the body, the mind—it's simply that whenever one does something, the other does something too. For instance, when your mind tells your right arm to raise, your body is simultaneously hearing this instruction. And when you raise this arm, you raise it both in your body and in your mind.

Obviously Leibnitz saw these two clocks as a spiritual metaphor, albeit, he was said to have believed quite strongly in a personal God—in a God with personal attributes. At the same time, considering how this story parallels the two brains theory—that we have two brains, each of which has their own sense of time—it appears there may have been more than God to what Leibnitz thought.

Of course, I'm not saying here that God the watchmaker actually sets these two clocks in perfect sync. I'm not even saying these two brains stay in sync. Still, can you see how what Leibnitz is saying—that time is the one thing which can simultaneously affect things with and without extension—so remarkably reflects our nature. And how it explains what we sense psychologically—that our two brains have separate clocks?

To some, what I've just said—that time is what connects the mind and body—may also sound like metaphysical mumbo jumbo. If so, then I suggest you reread the previous section on the two brains, or perhaps delve into it more deeply on your own. We are, after all, talking about observable and testable parallels in physiology and psychology.

And if you still find this hard to swallow? Then you should know I intend to discuss this idea further before the chapter ends. Hopefully, I'll address your concerns then.

Summing Up What We've Said So Far

So what have we heard so far? Three things.

First, Descartes says that our world is made up of two different substances. These two substances, which he called substances with and without extension, are what we now call matter and energy. He says that it's our experiences of these two substances that lead to our perceptions of the mind and body.

Spinoza then agrees, but says that what lies beneath these two perceptions is not two substances, but rather, one substance—a single material continuum which we sometimes experience mentally, as energy, and sometimes physically, as matter. Sort of reminiscent of how $e=mc^2$ treats energy and matter, don't you think?

Finally, Leibnitz adds that it's the timing of our perceptions which makes us feel that our mind and body connect. In essence, he says that what connects the mind and body psychologically is the timeline on which our life stories occur. Oddly, this parallels what physicists refer to as Minkowski's *spacetime*—the idea that space and time (and hence, all stories) are really four dimensions of one indissoluble whole (from the beginning part of Minkowski's address to the 80th Assembly of German Natural Scientists and Physicians, September 21, 1908).

Finding Mind Body Connections in the Composite Drawing

Now let's look at how these three ideas come together in our composite drawing. Can you find in Descartes' two substances, Leibnitz's two little clocks, each of which symbolizes one of the two ways we sense time—as *one-moment-at-a-time* (the body's sense of time), and as *time-over-time* (the mind's sense of time)? Can you also see how there are no clocks in Spinoza's continuum. Spiritual things feel timeless, remember?

Now see if you can find all the mind body dualities and mind body unities these three philosophical viewpoints create. Here, I strongly advise that you take your time, as it's easy to get lost and or drown in data.

Let's begin with the most obvious part—with Descartes' *two substances*—mind and body. Here, the thing to notice is how the mind takes up space, while the body does not. Obviously, this is a duality.

Now juxtapose this pair of complementary opposites to Spinoza's *continuum-of-substance*. This time, the thing to notice is how Descartes' two substances and Spinoza's one continuum form a tritinuum, a duality opposed to a unity.

Now add in Leibnitz's pair of clocks. Here, a second pair of complementary opposites—*one-moment-at-a-time;* the body's sense of time, and *time-over-time*; the mind's sense of time—form another mind body duality.

Now juxtapose this pair of opposites to Spinoza's continuum-of-substance. Here, the thing to see is how Leibnitz's two clocks and Spinoza's continuum of timelessness form a second tritinuum.

Now consider how these last two viewpoints form yet another mind body duality. Here, our mind's experience of physical reality; Spinoza's continuum-of-substance as a function of psychology—and our body's experience of the mental reality; Leibnitz's continuum-of-time as function of physics—form yet another pair of complementary opposites—mind body physics to mind body psychology.

Okay. Have I just drowned you in data? Sorry. I get excited when I'm discovering connections. And in truth, these are but a few of the myriad possible mind body dualities and unities present in these three viewpoints.

Fortunately, you don't need to know any of this to find your personal truth. You just need get a feel for how seamlessly these explanations integrate with one another. Indeed, this feeling is the main thing to come away with here, as it so accurately replicates what it's like to have a mind and a body.

As for reneging on my promise to not put you through any head-deadening philosophy, please realize that the four wise men get to me too. God forbid I leave one of them out. Out come the red hot pokers. Speaking of which, it's probably time for me to introduce our fourth and final philosopher, the one who is representing the rationalist wise man. Hopefully this fourth explanation will reveal what's kept us from putting all this together before.

Know this explanation is the easiest of all to understand. Even so, you should probably get ready to duck again. The fans are still on.

The Solution Hides in Plain Sight—Herbart's Contribution

Few people today have heard of our fourth and final philosopher. Yet he originated the idea of a dynamic unconscious some seventy years before

Freud. He also developed a method of teaching wherein teachers were expected to get students to personally connect to what they were learning, this at a time when children were expected to ingest and regurgitate what was being taught without comment. Not that it's so different for today's students, perhaps, in part because so few people today know of Herbart's work.

As for the mind body mystery, Herbart didn't posit much. Clearly, he favored the mind though, as even a cursory read of his work shows his primary focus was on ideas and on how they come into our awareness. To do this, he took Leibnitz's seminal conceptualization of the unconscious and expanded it into a description of how the mind works, beginning with that we have a dynamic threshold of awareness—above which we perceive things, and below which we do not.

Realize that today, we take for granted that things go on in us which we can't see, the things which in this book amount to the ever-present chatter of the four wise men. But it wasn't always so. For most of history, the idea of the unconscious didn't exist. Thus Herbart's threshold of perception was a significant step toward knowing the wise men exist.

Herbart called this threshold, a *limen*, a word which still exists as the root of the word, *subliminal*, as in subliminal suggestions. Equally interesting is the idea that while most ordinary folks believe we have an unconscious, many modern theorists deny this. To me, this is odd, since there's so much proof for that we respond to subliminal suggestions, an obvious nod to that we have things going on below our threshold of perception.

Herbart's Threshold as the Key to the Mind Body Mystery

Of course, the point for telling you all this is that, when Herbart talks about a threshold, he is supplying the key to the mind body mystery—the explanation for why we can't directly perceive the mind body connection. And yes, Herbart himself never refers to this threshold as a mind body element. However, when he describes ideas as separate entities above this threshold and a single mass below this threshold, he clearly anticipates the idea that we perceive mind and body above this threshold as two separate and distinct substances and below it as one continuum of substance.

Moreover, when we add his dynamic threshold of perception to our visual composite, the following becomes obvious. Descartes is correct above this threshold. Spinoza is correct below this threshold. Leibnitz is correct along this threshold. And Herbart explains why we haven't seen this before.

To wit, above the threshold, we perceive the mind and body as two separate and distinct substances—as the *two-sides-of-the-coin* view. This view, wherein you define the parts of things, is the materialist wise man's view. At the same time, we also know we are the being perceiving these two sides. Thus it logically follows that what we perceive as two separate experiences above the threshold is actually two attributes of one and the same experience below the threshold—the spiritual wise man's perspective; the *one-coin* view.

If we now add in Leibnitz's perspective, we see that both these ideas are true. We know this because these two perceptions change in recognizable patterns over time. Here, Leibnitz describes these changes perfectly when he uses a favorite idea of the rationalist wise man—time—and says that the mind and body each have their own sense of time. Thus Leibnitz accounts for how we psychologically experience these two viewpoints. Sometimes, we experience them as Descartes' two substances, and sometimes as Spinoza's two attributes of the same thing, "now perceived under the attribute of the mind, and now perceived under the attribute of the body." (*Ethics*, Baruch de Spinoza, The Hague, 1677).

This said, we are still faced with a tough question. If all three viewpoints are simultaneously true, then why can't we perceive them as a single truth?

Here, Herbart enters the fray. He explains that for the most part, all we're able to perceive is the separateness inherent in our world, body separate from mind, and vice versa. However, we also have a threshold of perception. And above this threshold, we perceive the mind and body as two separate things, while below this threshold, we cannot know but can logically assert the mind and body are one and the same.

This means, below this threshold is where the mind and body connect. Hence, our inability to see this connection.

Not coincidentally, this in many ways mirrors Descartes' idea that things are either clear and distinct, or unknowable. Here, the things we can perceive are analogous to what we can clearly and distinctly know and see in life; the stuff above the threshold. And the things we cannot see are analogous to the things which remain unknowable in life; the stuff below the threshold.

How Can We Be Sure the Mind and Body Connect?

How can we know for sure that the mind and body connect below our normal level of perception? Here, the answer somewhat resembles what happens when lakes dry up. I saw this happen once during a drought when I was a kid. The lake we used to fish in close-to dried up, and we were amazed to see all the lost fishing rods and reels which had been hiding at the bottom of the lake.

Something similar happens when we play a sport and feel like we're in the zone—or play or sing music and feel we're in the groove—or when we're writing or thinking and things just come to us—or when we feel a spiritual connection to anything or anyone. In these times, our threshold of perception drops low enough for us to sense the underlying reality. And when this happens, we see that Spinoza was indeed right. The mind and body truly are aspects of the one, all-encompassing all.

Of course, the best times to witness this connection occur in the moments wherein you have an aha. In these special moments, you feel amazed by how all things, including body and mind, connect. You also get to see the part of human nature which normally prevents you from seeing this truth—your tendency to trust only that part of your personal truth which rises above your threshold of consciousness.

In the moments wherein your threshold is lowered, however, you see all three views as true. As well as why you normally don't see things this way. Thus Herbart, while being far less known than the other three philosophers, ends up supplying the key element in the mind body mystery, as it literally explains why we believe in the four wise men.

Personal Time vs Science Teachers' Time

Before we explore the pragmatic tests which corroborate all this, I first need to expand a bit on how I am defining personal time. As opposed to how science teachers define time. Know we'll not be delving into the hideously complex philosophical nature of time. Nor will we be looking to mathematically or logically define time either. Rather we'll be looking only at what is absolutely necessary in order to discern personal time from science teachers' time. So if I say something which sounds less than scientific, bite your tongue. We're talking personal truth here.

Difference #1—How We Measure Time

To begin with, we measure time differently than science teachers do. Personal time is a rough quantity, whereas science teachers' measurements are more precise. To wit, personal time involves only our estimates of when things happen, how quickly or slowly, and how long they last. We'll call these things—*personal age*, e.g. yesterday, about a month ago, when I was a kid, before I was born—*personal rate*, e.g. dragging on, freaking slow, quick as a fox, fast as hell, faster than a speeding bullet—and *personal duration*, e.g. a New York minute, too bloody long, day and night, a dog's age, happily-ever-after.

Science teachers' time, however, involves standard scales and is more about precisely defining the timing of when things happen in different geographic locations, how frequently they happen, and for how long. We'll call these things—*calendrical reference*, e.g. March 23, 2006 at 1:15 PM EST, 810 A.D., Jurassic Period, Mesozoic Epoch—*temporal frequency*, e.g. 20 mph, 440 cycles per second, 90 BPM, 2800 rpm—and *chronological duration*, e.g. milliseconds, hours, days, light years.

So is this difference—that science teachers use standard scales to measure time, whereas we do not—the main difference? In one sense, yes, it is. Making personal guesses about time is a lot different than employing scientific instruments. Or even Rolex watches. However, an equally important difference has to do with our ability to experience these two kinds of time. With personal time, life passes at vague and often barely discernible rates, and rarely will two people agree on how long things last. Here, minutes can seem like hours and days like minutes. With science teachers' time, however, life passes at a more mechanistically constant pace. Two minutes are two minutes, no matter what is happening to us and regardless of who is saying this.

What accounts for this difference in how we measure time? In large part, it comes down to how time plays out on the horizontal axis. Here, one kind of time; science teachers' time, is true only in theory, while the other kind; personal time, is true only in the real world.

This difference then explains why it's so hard to personally connect to things we measure in standard scales, as well as why psychometric scales using everyday words don't translate well into theory. Personal scales, such as psychometric scales, exist only in the real world. Standard scales, such as those scientists use, exist only in theory.

Then there is how the vertical axis affects our perception of time. Here, your mind and body can logically know—and factually measure—science teachers' time. But only in theory. Whereas your mind and body can feel and tell stories about personal time. But only in the real world.

If you add these things together, what you find is that, in theory, time is pretty much what science teachers say it is—an unchanging, forward moving, logically linear progression through measurable increments.

Whereas, in the real world, time feels more like a constantly-evolving adventure story replete with edits and ongoing changes.

Perhaps this is why the scales scientists make their measurements with often resemble old fashioned, wooden rulers? Whereas, the personal guesstimates and descriptive impressions we make more resemble measurements made with children's toy rubber-rulers?

Difference #2—Where We Measure Time

A second important distinction between personal time and science teachers' time lies in how we define the past, present, and future. The difference lies in whether you think time passes at the same rate everywhere. Or not. With personal time, we intuitively sense that clocks register the same universal time regardless of where you are. Here, the past has already happened, the present is what's happening now, and the future has yet to be decided. But with science teachers' time, clocks in different places may literally run at different rates. Here, what's past, present, and future depend on where you are measuring time.

Now before you crash and burn, realize, we're only talking about two things here. One—what determines the past, present, and future—and two, inertial frames of reference. What the heck are *inertial frames of reference*?

Essentially, they're how science teachers refer to the place you are currently at—the boat, train, plane, car, rocket ship, or planet on which you're currently traveling. So, for instance, imagine you're traveling on a fast moving train, moreover, that this train is currently passing a train-station platform. Imagine, too, that your best friend is standing on this platform.

Now imagine that you look out the window at your friend standing on the platform. Can you picture him waving to you, and at the same time, see the window frame you're looking out of?

Despite what you know to be true logically, if you picture this, the more you focus on your friend, the more you'll feel that you are the one moving, and he is the one standing still. Alternately, the more you focus on the window frame, the more you'll feel like your friend is the one moving, and you are the one standing still. He'll even appear to be moving backwards with respect to you and your train.

Now imagine you switch places with your friend. This time, you are standing on the platform and your friend is on the train.

Can you picture him waving to you as the train passes the station?

So now, who is moving, and who is standing still?

From your personal perspective, nothing's changed. Your friend is still moving and you are still. However, your personal experience will now agree with the science teachers' truth, at least, as far as who is actually moving.

We call these changes in perspective, *Galilean Relativity*, something Einstein expanded on centuries later to arrive at special relativity. In essence, Galilean Relativity refers to the idea that the laws of physics are the same *within* inertial frames of reference. Smoke still rises straight up both on the platform and inside the moving train. But when we're in one frame of reference, and we're watching what's happening in another frame of reference, the laws of physics appear to change. Hence, the personal vs the science teachers' viewpoints as far as where we're measuring time.

This means there are actually two kinds of inertial frames of reference—the kind we sense; the personal kind—and kind science teachers measure; the physical kind. We derive ours from internally noticing where we are in relation to other external things, for instance, noticing we're on a moving train versus on a train station platform. Science teachers get theirs from noticing how fast things move with relation to each other, for instance, being on a rocket ship rapidly accelerating away from a planet versus being on this planet.

With personal frames of reference, then, sensing movement—even at relatively small scales—can often alter our experience of time. This happens each time we notice where we are, while also noticing something moving differently from us—something outside of our personal frame of reference. For instance, if we look out at our friend waving to us from the train station platform while we're noticing the window frame from inside a moving train—we'll feel like time is passing differently in these two places.

With physical frames of reference, however, measuring movement at the scale of people on trains and people on train-station platforms changes nothing with regard to time. So to science teachers, we and the moving trains both exist within the same inertial frame of reference. And because changes in position and momentum at this scale don't measurably alter the laws of physics, they don't alter clocks. Thus, to science teachers, time stays the same.

Have I lost you? If so, please know, you're not alone. I, myself, find this stuff incredibly hard to understand, let alone, to explain. Moreover, if I could, I'd sidestep it entirely. But in a book which focuses on time as what creates our sense of mind and body, this would be impossible.

Know that in Book III, chapter eight, *Uncertainty & Prediction—a Human Obsession*, I'll offer a much better explanation. There, we'll be looking at how inertial frames of reference prove that there are things both we and the science teachers cannot know. Hopefully, this will help.

This said, the main thing to come away with here is that with personal time, our focus is on how we feel and talk about time passing—whereas with science teachers' time, the focus is on how they measure and conceptualize time passing. Moreover, while our intuitive sense of time can change based on whether we sense we are moving or not, out there, time always moves at a steady speed. Well, almost always.

Difference #3—How Quickly Time Passes

As I'm sure you realize by now, when it comes to the four wise men, there's never an end to their madness. To wit, as if they haven't already screwed with your head enough, there's a second kind of relativity which affects our sense of time. Here, we add the idea that light moves at the same speed regardless of which inertial frame of reference you are in. We call this kind of relativity, *special* relativity, in that it applies Einstein's principles of relativity only to special cases—to inertial frames of reference.

What exactly does this change with regard to our sense of time?

Personally? Not much. But according to science teachers, if we travel at very fast speeds—at or near the speed of light—by changing where we are in space, we physically change where we are in time, at least with reference to someone else who is moving much more slowly.

Thus, according to science teachers, if you circle the Earth backwards in a fast jet, time in the jet will literally pass at a different rate than time on the ground. Amazingly, in 1972, Joseph Hafele and Richard Keating proved this to be true. They found that clocks in a high speed jet lost about 59 nanoseconds while flying eastward with regard to the Earth, and gained 273 nanoseconds while flying westwards (*Introducing Time*, C. Callender, R. Edney, Icon Books Ltd, London).

Did you get that? For the clocks in these planes and the clocks on the ground, time literally passed at different rates. And no, there was nothing wrong with the clocks. The relative differences between inertial frames of reference included differences in the rate at which time passed.

According to special relativity, then, if there is a significant speed difference between two inertial frames of reference, then the rate at which time passes within these frames will be different. Moving faster relative to another frame will cause time to dilate and slow down. And moving slower will cause time to contract and speed up.

Of course, we'll feel no change at all within our current frame of reference. Certainly, no one in Hafele and Keating's experiment felt time change. But they literally measured a change in the rate at which time passed. Thus, in these kinds of situations, what is out there changes, while what we feel does not.

What's the big deal, you say? Well if you were to compare your experience of time to that of folks on a distant planet, the same moment can be in your future and in another person's past. And no, you did not just read that wrong. Special relativity not only describes how time can pass at different rates in different places. It also describes how what is past, present, and future change depending on where you are.

For instance, consider how star light relates to time. We're told, and most of us have no trouble imagining, that the star light we see today began traveling toward us millions of light years ago.

So the question is, to what time does the light reaching us today refer? To the past? To the present? To the future?

Surprisingly, the answer depends on the speed at which you are moving in relation to this light. To the inhabitants of a planet near that distant star, the light reaching us today is occurring in their future and in our present. But while we both would agree that this is occurring in our present, to us, this light is coming from their past.

What if we were in a very fast rocket ship traveling back toward this star? Would this take us back in time?

As you might guess, this depends on whose perspective you're referring to. With regard to the star light reaching Earth, yes, it will. But with regard to our space ship, no it won't. And with regard to the inhabitants of a planet near that star, we'd be moving closer to their present.

Have I lost you again? Don't give it another thought. Most people have trouble understanding time. Including me. The trouble, of course, is that we've been convinced by the four ninnies that we must reconcile personal time with science teachers' time. In truth, there appears to be no end to the confusion these bozos can inflict on us, including the biggest one of all with regard to time—whether the future is already written within the light that reaches us, or whether we can change this future.

Fortunately, we need not answer these questions to arrive at a personal truth. We need only remember that personal truth is not a universal truth. Rather, it's a relative truth. This means your sense of what's past, present, and future resets each time you notice where you are. And it also depends on how fast you're moving relative to other places. Hence each change in your position and momentum initiates another round of personal time. At least if you're moving in a relatively straight line at a close to steady speed—such as when you're moving in a train, plane, boat, on a planet, or in a rocket ship.

Difference #4—Whether Space and Time Are Separate

Then there's the idea that, to us, time and space are two different things and we talk about them separately. But to science teachers, space and time are two aspects of one thing—*spacetime*—and you can't talk about one without the other. Thus, to us, space is where things happen and time is how fast and for how long, whereas to science teachers, spacetime is where things happen and time is more like geography than chronology.

Confusing, isn't it? Don't worry. If you apply the five aspects we learned about in the last chapter, it's simpler than it appears.

Begin with this. To us, space and time are a duality—two separate things. Here, space and time are like two sides of a coin (first aspect). Whereas to science teachers, space and time are two attributes of one and the same thing. And together, these two attributes make one coin—the unity of spacetime (second aspect).

At the same time, while we can know with certainty that both ways of seeing time are simultaneously true, we can never actually see them both as true at the same time (third aspect). The fourth aspect explains why. Because sums add differently in theory and in the real world, adding space and time result in two different views.

Thus according to the fourth aspect, in theory, we can conceptualize spacetime as four dimensional geography or even as eleven dimensional strings. But in the real world, seeing three dimensions change over time is our limit. This, in part, is why we experience space and time as being separate. In effect, this allows us to experience all four dimensions personally.

Beyond this limit, though, our real world efforts fall apart. At least until we remember the fifth aspect, wherein we're told that despite our limited visual abilities, we can indeed personally experience truths which exceed our four dimensional limit. This happens whenever we experience something which lowers our threshold of perception. Moreover, there's only one thing you really need to see here—that the two ways we see time are mirrored in how the mind experiences time differently than the body.

Ultimately, this means that to truly know the mind and body, we must see our two experiences of time as a pair of complementary opposites. On one side, we have *one-moment-at-a-time*, the body's way of sensing time. And on the other, we have *time-over-time*, the mind's way of sensing time. Moreover, while this seems to yet again confirm our hypothesis—that mind and body exist as separate but interactive experiences—we still need to find ways in which to reliably test this in real life situations. This is what we'll look at next.

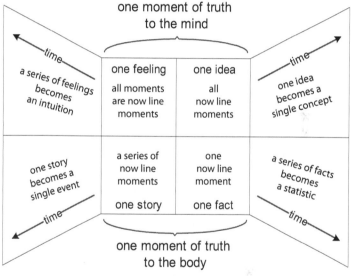

Ms. Goodmind versus Mr. Hardbody
(How Time Creates the Two Core Personality Experiences:
Thoughts and Impressions)
(© 2007 Steven Paglierani   The Center for Emergence)

A
Thought

one moment of truth
to the mind

one feeling	one idea
all moments are now line moments	all now line moments
a series of now line moments	one now line moment
one story	one fact

a series of feelings becomes an intuition

one idea becomes a single concept

one story becomes a single event

a series of facts becomes a statistic

one moment of truth
to the body

An
Impression

Mind Time & Body Time—The Two Kinds of Personal Time

What are these two senses of personal time like?

To the mind's brain, the world is made up of sensible sequences of experience. Slice it up and put it in order and you find the truth. But to the body's brain, dividing things into sensible sequences only leads to confusion. Thus it's the physical experience of the whole thing that matters. Truth lies in what something is, not in what something does.

Confused? Then take a look at the composite drawing on the previous page, the one I've titled *Ms. Goodmind versus Mr. Hardbody (how time creates the two core personality experiences: thoughts and impressions)*. Here you'll find the four wise men have divided themselves into two opposing groups—a mind based group, and a body based group. You'll also find two little characters who are the spokespersons for these two groups—Ms. Goodmind, and Mr. Hardbody.

So what do you think? Do they appear trite and cartoonish? In reality, they're anything but. In fact, these two characters represent the two most significant qualities in human personality—mind and body. In this way, they have a lot to tell you about all human beings, including yourself. Indeed, one of these two beings is even a lot like you. Either you are like Ms. Goodmind, a *mind first* person—or like Mr. Hardbody, a *body first* person.

Know we'll delve more into what all this means in a moment, and in the next book, we'll explore this topic in depth. For now though, we're going to focus only on how you can use personal time to know which of these two types of people you are—a mind first person or a body first person. Can you guess yet which one you are? You're about to find out.

The Mind First State vs The Body First State

Let's start by looking at the drawing I've placed at the top of the opposite page, the one titled *Mind First State*. In it, you'll find the typical mind body state for a mind first person. Notice, first, the two waves of experience—the bigger one on the left which represents the mind, and the smaller one on the right which represents the body.

Now look closer and you'll notice the two little clocks which have been embedded in these waves, each representing a kind of time. Here, the wave of thought experience is significantly larger than the wave of impression experience. Thus this person senses time mainly as *time over time*.

Now compare this drawing to the one I've placed at the bottom of this page, the one titled, *Body First State*. Can you see how the size of the waves and thus, this person's awareness of time, is the reverse of the

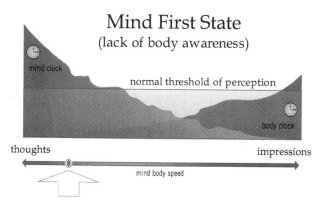

Mind First State
(lack of body awareness)

previous person's? Here we see the typical mind body state of a body first person, including that the way this person normally senses time is as *one-moment-at-a-time*, rather than as *time-over-time*.

Now consider how this difference could be used as the basis for a series of pragmatic tests to determine your mind body preference—whether you are a mind first person, or a body first person. This is what the tests in the next section are based on—on the mind's sense of time versus the body's sense of time.

Want to make this a bit easier on yourself? Then try calling the body's sense of time, *simple time*, and the mind's, *complex time*, a nod to that they're both ideas. Here, simple time refers to the way the body senses time, as individual points in time. Whereas complex time refers to the way the mind senses time, as sequences of points in time. Interestingly enough, this gives us yet another clue as to our mind-body orientation—how we gauge success and failure. Meaning what exactly? Let's see.

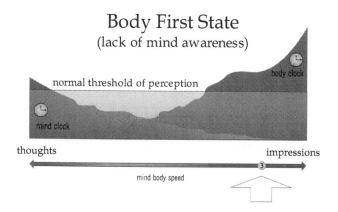

Body First State
(lack of mind awareness)

How Time Affects Our Sense of Success and Failure

For many of us, success and failure seems to depend on how well we analyze the past. However, not all people feel this way. Thus while mind first people tend to rate success and failure based on past performance, body first people tend to see success and failure as more of a measure of how you're doing in the present.

I mention this as it highlights a good way to identify people's mind-body orientation. And their default sense of time. To wit, to mind first folks, life has a past, present, and future. But to body first folks, life occurs only in the present. Thus if you're mind first, you'll experience each success and failure in complex time. Whereas if you're body first, you'll experience each success and failure in simple time.

What does this mean?

If you're a mind first person, you'll tend to analyze your successes or failures, then assign them to categories. Thus mind first people focus more on frequency—how often these events happen. But if you're a body first person, each success or failure will feel like it's the only success or failure you've had. Thus body first people focus more on how intense each event is.

This difference—frequency or intensity—gives you a good way to know whether you're experiencing simple time or complex time. When you make a decision based on how intense something feels, it's likely you're experiencing simple time—the body's sense of time. But when you make a decision based on how often something happens, it's likely you're experiencing complex time—the mind's sense of time.

Why Single Events Feel Intense

Does this intensity thing sound counterintuitive? It is. You'd think that experiencing multiple events would feel more intense, not less. However, were you to recall a time wherein you felt something intensely, say, a time when your little angel dropped a glass of milk on a newly waxed kitchen floor, you'd find that in those moments, it didn't matter whether it was the first time or the fiftieth time. All you felt was, "NOT AGAIN!"

If you were to then plan a camping trip, however, and needed to figure out how many glasses you'd need to bring, you might find it hard to focus on anything but frequency. Here, your primary concern would likely shift away from how bad it feels when your child drops a glass and onto how often your little earthly representative of Shiva does this.

How Your Mind Body State Affects Your Taste in Music

Yet one more way to get a feel for this difference is to compare the two ways we sense time to the bass and treble controls on a stereo. To wit, when you're listening to music and your body is in charge, physically feeling the bass is what's important. So you crank up the volume, especially the lows. But when you're listening to music and your mind is in charge, hearing crystal clear highs is what's important. So you listen at a lower volume so you can mentally notice more detail.

Not coincidentally, were you to pay attention to your sense of time in these two situations, you'd notice that the more you focus on the low frequencies, the more time seems to slow down, whereas the more you focus on the high frequencies, the faster time seems to pass. Here we see yet another nod to how the frequency of what we sense—in this case the frequency of the sound—determines which of our brains processes it.

Overall, the thing to see here is how we can use the two ways we sense time to create a series of simple tests wherein we can know which brain is in charge. And at this point, rather than put you through any more mind-deadening theory, let's just try this on for size.

We'll begin with a brief look at the test conditions—followed by some typical tests.

Testing For Your Mind-Body Orientation

When I think back on all the things I went through to come up with some usable mind-body orientation tests, I am reminded of how erratic and convoluted the discovery process can be. And how simple it can seem in hindsight. For instance, why didn't I see as good tests what I had done with Audrey—to sing and tap time, or with Lori—to speak and draw? They are both excellent tests. This makes me wonder how "throwing fives" became my first test. This said, the thing to keep in mind here is what all these tests have in common—the question—which comes first, the mind or the body?

What exactly should you be looking for? Start with this.

Like all truths, mind-body orientation lies on a continuum between two complementary opposites. Here, the essence of these two end points is which comes first, your mind's experience or your body's. This is why, when I titled Audrey's section, I described her as a *mind-before-body* person. And when I wrote about Lori, I referred to her as a *body-before-mind* person.

In my everyday life, when I refer to these two experiences, I generally shorten these phrases to *mind first* and *body first*. Moreover, what I'm looking for in all these tests is a clear and distinct observation which tells me which of these two theoretical orientations best describes a person's norm.

Why a theoretical norm? Because as I've said previously, mind-body orientation is like handedness. In theory, we're either right or left handed. But in the real world, we're mixes of both. Mind-body orientation is similar, in that we tend toward one of these styles. But we also have what I call mind body *counter preferences,* patterns of exceptions wherein our orientation reverses for no apparent reason.

What we're looking for in these tests then is some sort of personal norm with regard to the mind and body, a personal tendency as to which comes first—the mind or body—in a series of real life situations.

In addition, in order for these results to be useful, they must consistently result in the same mind-body orientation, including that these results must be confirmed through countertests as falsifiable. Here, deliberately inverting the test outcomes so as to favor the opposite orientation should make the person feel observably uncomfortable.

As for the tests I'm about to describe, know they are meant only as a starting point from which to develop your own tests. What you're looking to learn here then is not these particular tests, per se. Rather, you're looking to learn the concept on which all these tests are based—how time affects the mind differently than the body.

In addition, to become proficient at administering these tests, you must have a clear and distinct sense of your own mind-body orientation. This should include, at minimum, several counter preferences. For example, in my case, I am a mind first person. But when I sing and don't notice the meaning of the words—dance and physically feel more than hear the music—and engineer recording sessions entirely from my fingers, I am clearly exhibiting body first counter preferences.

Now let's explore a few of the actual tests, beginning with the one I mentioned as being my first mind-body orientation test; "throwing fives."

Four Mind-Body Orientation Tests

Before you administer these tests, there are a few things to keep in mind. If people mentally prepare before doing a test, this will invalidate the results. This makes learning to see people doing this—and having ways to get them to stop doing this—an absolute necessity.

Be aware then that the less people think before responding, the more valid the test result. Thus a good thing to include in your pre-test instructions is a request that people respond to your requests as quickly as possible and without thinking.

In addition, in order to confidently interpret the results of these tests, you must have gotten clear results when you did them on yourself. Also, you need to be careful not to logically assume how a test will turn out, as this will likely skew what you see.

Now the tests.

Mind-Body Orientation Test #1—Throwing Fives

Like all mind-body orientation tests, this one is relatively simple. You ask the person to do the following.

Without thinking and as quickly as possible, fully extend an arm—palm face forward, and with all five fingers spread apart—while simultaneously saying the word *five*. Can you picture someone doing this?

Try it. Stand up. Now as fast as you can and without thinking extend an arm—palm face forward—as if you are signaling someone to stop. At the same time, say the word five out loud.

What will happen? Either your arm, hand, and fingers will begin to extend before you start saying the word *five*—or you'll start saying *five* before your arm, hand, and fingers begin to extend.

Did your hand start first? Then your normal mind-body orientation is body first. Did you say the word *five* first? Then your normal orientation is mind first.

Know I've seen people so mentally control themselves that the outcome is repeatedly invalid. Here, you'll likely observe people mentally preparing, rather than following the part of the instructions which ask them to do this as quickly as possible and without thinking.

If this happens, you can compensate for this by asking people to deliberately cause one action to begin before the other. Either they must have their arm begin to extend before they start saying the word *five*—or they must say the word *five* before their arm begin to extend. Moreover, there must be no observable prep time spent inbetween doing these two acts. If there is, here again, the results will be invalid.

What are you looking for this time? Essentially, for which outcome is easier to reach. In other words, does this person find it easier to begin to extend an arm before starting to say the word *five*? Or does this person find it easier to say the word *five* before beginning to extend an arm? If the former, then this person is body first. And if the later, then this person is mind first.

Would you like to improve your ability to administer this test? Then practice deliberately arriving at both of these outcomes yourself. Deliberately have your hand start extending first. Then deliberately say the word *five* before your arm begins to extend. If you do, you'll be surprised at how this simple exercise can improve your sense of the two mind-body orientations, including your ability to see these two orientations in others.

Mind-Body Orientation Test #2—the Draw and Speak Test

Have you ever had to give someone directions? This test looks at which comes first, the drawn map or the spoken words. Thus all you need do here is ask the person to draw the roads while describing the drive. If the drawing is occurring ahead of the words, then the person is body first. And if the words get spoken ahead of the drawing, then the person is mind first.

Again, a good way to validate the test is to ask people to reverse their normal order, then watch for discomfort and disorientation. If they normally draw then speak, ask them to speak first, then draw. And if they normally speak then draw, then ask them to draw then speak.

What if the results of a test contradict a previous test, the throwing fives test, for instance?

If this happens, don't be alarmed. One of these tests represents their norm, and the other, a counter preference. Indeed, finding people's counter preferences is a good long term goal, as it literally teaches people to see options they normally don't consider. Thus, if this happens, make a note of it, and just go on to another test.

Mind-Body Orientation Test #3—the Sing and Tap Test

For the less inhibited, singing or humming while tapping a hand on their leg is also a good test. As is singing or humming while snapping their fingers. Know it usually doesn't matter much whether people sit or stand. All that matters is that you witness a clear preference for which comes first, the singing / humming, or the tapping / snapping.

Here again, asking people to deliberately reverse this outcome gives you a method with which to arrive at a false outcome, and doing this can validate the results. Moreover, once you've done these tests a few times, you'll realize how easy it is to get clear and distinct results. Mind-body orientations are literally this obvious.

Mind-Body Orientation Test #4—the Ultimate Test: Slow Talking

This last test is my favorite, as it's nearly impossible to fake the results. It's also one of the easiest tests to administer and gives accurate results. I usually use it in all first sessions with couples, as well as with anyone whom identifies as having ADHD. It's also a good test for determining the severity of someone's Asperger's, as well as for one's general vulnerability to overeating.

Here's all you do.

With both of you sitting, or with both of you standing, say something to this person at an exaggeratedly slow pace. What should you say? It doesn't matter really, albeit, simple is better.

For instance, you could say to this person, "How ... do ... you ... feel ... when ... people ... talk ... this ... slowly?" Or, "Do... you ... ever ... get ... annoyed ... when ... people ... talk ... too quickly?"

When mind first people get spoken to like this, they go out of their minds. Literally. Slow talk makes them so aware of their body that it ruins their ability to think. Conversely, body first people love it when you talk this slow. Indeed, this will often make them smile, as hearing words at this pace brings what you're saying into focus.

How accurate is this test?

I once attended an all day seminar wherein one of my favorite neuro researchers was presenting on the brain. I respect this man a lot and see him as having done some particularly good original work on the relationship between neurotransmitters and hormones with regard to brain functioning. He literally discovered a fractal for this relationship. However, when I, at the end of his seminar, asked him to comment on the brain in the body (the enteric brain), his faced deadened and he became noticeably angry. At which point, he told everyone, "this question is easy to answer—there is no enteric brain."

Right after this, people began exiting the seminar, and as they did, I approached him to ask him to comment more. Moreover, as my work relies heavily on the existence of the enteric brain, I was feeling quite deflated. I then tried to dialogue with him about what made him so mad, and the more I tried to get him to comment, the more annoyed he got. At which point, I slow talked, rather loudly, to all the people still in room, that "this ... is ... what ... the ... non ... existent ... enteric ... brain ... feels ... like." Where upon every single person listening to our exchange, and everyone in the process of exiting—some hundred plus people actually—froze in surprise, including the neuro researcher. He and I then proceeded to have an entirely different conversation, the tone of which was now respectful and curious.

In another seminar—this one an Asperger's / Autism seminar being given by my one of my favorite speakers, John Ortiz—I was asked to briefly describe to the conference attendees my work on mind-body orientation. At which point, I slow talked a single sentence to a room of several hundred people, mainly professionals, with the same result. They all froze in surprise at how obvious the effect of this test was.

What makes me begin couples therapies with slow talk? Mainly, it's that most couples include one person of each orientation. One spouse will be mind first, and the other, body first. Here, the mind first spouse will usually see the body first spouse as being distant and unwilling to communicate, when in truth, body first people merely hear and speak words much differently than mind first people.

Remember too that we're talking about a relative difference here, not an absolute one. In other words, all I'm saying here is that, by comparison, one person is noticeably more mind orientated than the other.

What does this do to relationships? Misread, it causes people to feel unloved. Thus, often the body first spouse will give up after years of being accused of not trying to communicate—while the mind first spouse will look to the world like a critical control freak.

What happens when couples realize the truth? Usually, the body first person grins with delight, as he or she knows right away that someone hears them and speaks their language. Whereas the mind first person usually looks dazed and confused as, for the first time, they see evidence for there being a lot more to their spouse's lack of communication than that he or she just won't try. Or doesn't love them.

More on this in Book III.

The Mind and Body as Radio Stations

Lastly, we have one more thing to discuss before we end this chapter—how our mind-body orientation makes us vulnerable to the four wise men's nonsense. What I'm saying is, we literally derive our belief in the four wise men from our mind-body orientation. How does this happen? To see, we'll need to look at two things. First, we'll need to look at how our two brains function like two radio stations. Second, we'll need to look at how our listening habits lead to four possible brain processing patterns—the four viewpoints I've been calling the four wise men.

Let's begin by looking at the drawing on the opposite page, the one titled, *The Two Radio Receivers (the mind brain and the body brain)*. Here, you'll find four people, all lying down, each numbered with one of the quadrants of the wise men's map.

What does this drawing represent? To see, start by noticing how each person has what appear to be two radio station towers rising up out of them, one for the mind and one for the body. Know that like real life radio station towers, these two towers differ mainly in what frequencies they broadcast and receive. Here, the radio station tower in the head transmits and receives at a higher frequency than the radio station tower

The Two Radio Receivers
(the mind brain & the body brain)

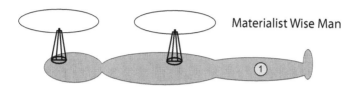

Materialist Wise Man

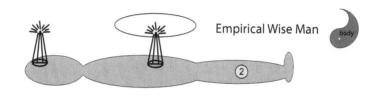

Empirical Wise Man

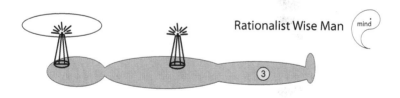

Rationalist Wise Man

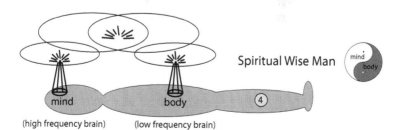

Spiritual Wise Man

(high frequency brain)   (low frequency brain)

in the gut. Hence the brain in the head is called the *high frequency brain*, and the brain in the gut, the *low frequency brain*.

This idea—that our two brains send and receive information at difference frequencies—is what underlies our belief in a separate mind and body. No coincidence, many spiritual belief systems, for instance, yoga philosophy, include references to that different frequencies affect different points on the spine (chakras), including the idea that the higher the frequency, the higher the affected part of the spine.

Modern yoga practitioners then add to this that there are colors associated to these points, moreover, that these colors also increase in frequency as you ascend the spine, from the slower frequencies of deep reds and oranges at the base of the spine to the faster frequencies of ultra violets and white at the crown of the head.

Here again, we see psychophysical parallels between the mind and body—between our mind's sense of the world and what science tells us is happening.

How the Transmit Waves and Receive Ovals Create the Self

Now look at the tops of the radio station towers. Can you see how some towers have both transmit waves and receive ovals and some only have one or the other. Here, the patterns of these transmit waves and receive ovals mirror the four ways we experience the self.

Thus, the materialist wise man's person shows no self awareness (no transmit waves, two sets of receive ovals). The empirical wise man's person shows only body self awareness (two sets of transmit waves, only a body oval). The rationalist wise man's person shows only mind self awareness (two sets of transmit waves, only a mind oval). And the spiritual wise man's person shows an extended self awareness (two sets of transmit waves and a combined mind body oval).

How They Also Create Our Sense of Personal Time

In addition, because our sense of personal time comes from noticing differences between our two brains, these four send-receive patterns explain why the four wise men sense time differently.

Here, the materialist wise man's two towers are both in receive only mode. Thus he senses no time differences. So to him, time is something external, a difference in what is changing "out there." Whereas the empirical wise man's body tower is in send and receive mode, while his mind tower is in send only mode. Thus he senses time differences in two ways—one, as the difference between what is physically "out there" and what is physically "in here," and two, as the differences between body reception and the lack of mind reception.

This is the exact opposite of the rationalist wise man's towers, wherein his mind tower is in send and receive mode while his body tower is in send only mode. Thus he senses time differences in two ways as well—one, as the difference between what is mentally "out there" and what is mentally "in here" and two, as the differences between mind reception and the lack of body reception. And finally, the spiritual wise man's towers are both in send and receive mode. Thus there are no differences to sense, neither between what is "out there" and what is "in here," nor between the mind and the body. Hence, the timelessness of the spiritual wise man's truth.

The main thing to see here, of course, is how our two brains function like two radio stations, each occupying it's own part of the electrochemical broadcast frequency band. Similar to how actual radio station programming varies from station to station (e.g. high energy versus easy listening), the programming in our two brains varies as well, with the high brow talk radio broadcasts on the mind brain network, and the sports and music broadcasts on the body brain network.

How Not Tuning-In to Others is the Main Problem

Now consider how different this idea is from the common belief that in order to communicate well with others, you need to learn the right words. Yes, there is definitely value in learning to use language better. But our problems with communication lie less in the words we use, and more in that we need to learn how to tune in to others.

Fortunately, there's only one thing you need to learn in order to do this. You need to learn to adjust the speed at which you communicate. By doing this, you can vastly improve your ability to hear, and connect, to people. Indeed, I recently read that body first physicist, Niels Bohr, once commented that you should, "never talk faster than you think." And when I read this, I suddenly understood volumes about what kept mind first folks like Einstein from following many of Bohr's discussions.

In Books II and III, we'll talk a lot more about how adjusting your broadcast frequency can change your life. For now, the thing to take away is twofold. One, there is physiological, psychological, empirical, and spiritual evidence for that there is a separate mind and body. Two, if you can use this knowledge to determine people's mind-body orientation, you can improve the quality of everything you do in life.

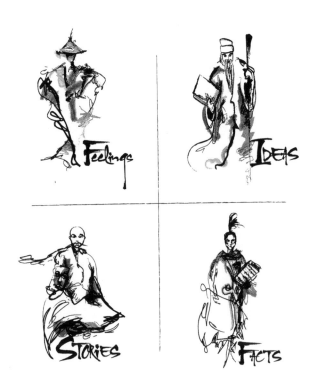

Notes Written in the Margins of Chapter Four

On My Choice to Use the Word *Impression*

Nowhere in this book did I deliberate longer than on which word to use for the opposite of *thoughts*. Part of my difficulty was that I have spent the better part of the decade prior to my discovery of the four wise men using the word *feelings* as the opposite of the word *thoughts*, including for my work in and around the mind body connection. This left me either with the unpleasant choice of finding a new word for the spiritual wise man's language, or with the unattractive prospect of having to revise the thousands of pages of existing text and diagrams I've already published on my Web site.

In the end, I opted for the later and chose to use the word *impressions* to represent the combined experience of facts and stories. In doing so, I let the spiritual wise man keep his word *feelings*. To my surprise, no sooner did I decide to do this than I began having more realizations as to what makes these two words exactly right for where they are.

For one thing, the more I thought about the word *impressions*, the more I realized, we already use this word this way in everything from the fact plus story "diagnostic impressions" of an M.D. and the "lost wax impressions" of bronze sculpture to the "good first impressions" of job interviews and "lasting impressions" of a great work of art. In every case, the word "impressions" refers to the impact something makes on something else. This can be anything from the impact walking in wet sand makes on you and the bad impression you make on your new girlfriend's parents to the lack of impression your final presentation makes on your history professor and the indent that the dent in your new red sports car puts in your mood.

The point, of course, in all these cases, is that facts and stories combine to leave a tangible, physical, life-shaped "imprint" in you—literally the impression any group of facts plus stories makes on you. Moreover, this happens because a substance without extension, e.g. your feelings about the dented car, makes an impression on something with extension—you. And since ideas and feelings both occur on the mind end of the vertical axis and as such, are both energies, this makes sense. Feelings and ideas are both thoughts, and thoughts can leave us with impressions. More proof that the mind and body interact.

Of course, this realization also refined my sense of what feelings are. Clearly, feelings are more the product of the mind seeking to identify something going on in the body than something as simple and incoherent as the idea of emotions. This is why, when we're asked what we are feeling, we generally look up, not down. We always look in the direction of where we expect to find answers. This is also is why, when we search our mind, we automatically look up, and when we search our body, we automatically look down. And given what we now know about the two brains and their different broadcast frequencies, this makes sense, does it not?

On Ryle's "Ghost in the Machine"

Before researching this chapter, I had not heard of Gilbert Ryle. Nor had I known of his book slamming Descartes. As I read him in his own words though, I was reminded of the lengths people will go to defend their wise man. To wit, to Ryle, the rationalist wise man seems the only sane choice, and anyone who disagrees with him is being patently absurd and mindlessly stupid.

In part, Ryle's weapon is something called *linguistic analysis*, a once admired though somewhat dated form of vitriolic rationalist ridicule wherein logic is used to turn a person's own words against them. Ironically, Ryle's reference to Descartes' dualism being the ghost in the machine, in part, led to my realization that ghosts, like the physicist's energy, are reified concepts, more the invisible man of physics being sprayed with water than a mysterious and ultimately non existent substance.

So what does this mean about ghosts being real?

If energy is a reified pattern of change in matter, and if someone's body is physically affected by seeing a ghost, then I guess they are. You can, after all, measure how these things affect people. Perhaps ghosts, minds, and energy have more in common than previously acknowledged?

On Cause Versus Correlation

Most of us take for granted the idea of cause and effect, and it's easy enough to see why. Like universal time, it seems intuitive. However, were you to ingest enough Hume and Berkeley, you'd realize that as far as the real world, we can neither directly see nor measure cause and effect (Hume), nor directly see or measure material reality (Berkeley). In truth, we base both these assumptions on rational and material interpretations of what we can see, including that what we can see is a literal reality, this despite the fact that both can be true only in theory.

What we can observe of course is that things occur in the same time and space. This includes things like the ingredients we put into a cake and how long we bake it.

So do these things account for how a cake tastes? If they did, then mass produced cakes would taste just as good as homemade cakes.

Do we have anything to gain from observing these facts then? Absolutely. But only if we remember that these facts cannot be the cause of the taste, as taste, like life itself, is an emergent quality.

On Success and the Gambler's Fallacy

When I was writing the subsection on how time affects our sesne of success and failure, I was reminded of something called *the gambler's fallacy*. Here, we are told that after a flipped coin comes up heads 99 times in a row, the odds it will come up heads in the next throw is still the same as in the first throw—fifty-fifty. I raise this as, even after years of being told this, my mind still has trouble wrapping itself around this idea. And yes, I know mentally it is true. But my gut just hasn't caught on yet. Another downside to being mind first perhaps.

The point is, mind first folks think success depends on what comes before it. But according to the gambler's fallacy, if discovery is truly an emergent quality, then success may have less to do with understanding the past and more to do with being consciously present.

Resources for Chapter Four—The Mind Body Mystery

On Time

Callender, C. and R. Edney. (2004). *Introducing Time*. London: Icon Books Ltd. (This company, Icon Books Ltd, publishes a whole series of books on complex topics wherein the visual descriptions balance well with the verbal explanations. And while they may, at first glance, appear to be simple overviews, they are deceptively simple and ultimately quite thorough. I highly recommend them.)

Howard, Don. (2008). *Albert Einstein: Physicist, Philosopher, Humanitarian*. Course 8122. Chantilly, VA: The Teaching Company. (Professor Howard is an expert on both Einstein's personal papers and his physics. And while I bought this selection based on what I assumed from the title, I ended up using some of what I learned in my descriptions of time. Be forewarned though. Professor Howard's a bit dry. Even so, he's well worth the effort.)

On the Mind Body Connection

Gershon, Dr. Michael D. (1998). *The Second Brain—Your Gut Has a Mind of Its Own*. New York: Harper Collins. (I cannot emphasize enough how important this book is. Moreover, should you have any doubt, Google the negative reactions to it. You'll find there are quite a few. This tells me Gershon's work must have much in the way of truth, as truths which challenge little to nothing usually generate little in the way of reaction, whereas truths which threaten less viable theories usually generate much resistance.)

Ryle, Gilbert. (2002, 1949). *The Concept of Mind*. Chicago: The University of Chicago Press. (As I've mentioned several times previously, I respect people who openly posit their truths. Thus while I thoroughly disagree with Ryle as to how human nature works, I so admire him for passionately voicing his beliefs.)

On the Four Philosophers

Herbart, J. F. (1877). *Possibility and Necessity of Applying Mathematics in Psychology*. Trans. from German by H. Haanel. First published in Journal of Speculative Philosophy, 11, 251-26. Baltimore, Maryland. (A brief article worth reading for his comments on how theory and the real world must connect.)

Magee, Brian. (2006). *The Story of Philosophy*. New York: Dorling Kindersley Limited, Barnes & Noble. (I was surprised by how good this book was. On the surface, it appeared to be just another compendium of the usual suspects. But right from the opening page, it grabbed my attention with less known stories and great connections. If you never read another general book on philosophy, this is the one to read. I highly recommend it.)

Kenny, Anthony. (2006). *A New History of Western Philosophy, The Rise of Modern Philosophy, Volume 3*, Oxford, UK: Clarendon Press.

Kenny, Anthony. (2006, 2001, 1994). *The Oxford Illustrated History of Western Philosophy*. New York: Oxford University Press. (Kenny's writing style is also a bit dry. Nevertheless, he offers solid background information.)

On The Unconscious

Papineau, David and Selina, Howard. (2005). *Introducing Consciousness.* London: Icon Books Ltd. (Another of Icon's thought provoking visual guides to a complex topic. Remember to go slow, though, as it's much deeper than a casual look makes it seem.)

Hebb, Donald Olding. (1980). *Essay on Mind.* Hillsdale, NJ: Lawrence Erlbaum Associates.

Montmasson, Joseph-Marie. (1999). *Invention and the Unconscious.* Trans. with a preface by H. Stafford Hatfield. New York: Routledge.

Banerjee, J. C. (1994). *Encyclopaedic Dictionary of Psychological Terms.* New Delhi, India: M.D. Publications Pvt. Ltd.

Singh, Arun Kumar. (1991). *The Comprehensive History of Psychology.* New Delhi, India: Motilal Banarsidass Publishers.

Odds and Ends

Fleck, Ludwik. (1935). *The Genesis and Development of a Scientific Fact.* English translation edited by T.J. Trenn and R.K. Merton. (1979). foreword by Thomas Kuhn. Chicago: University of Chicago Press. (This brilliant work by a Polish scientist raises some excellent points about the nature of truth in science. In fact, one of Fleck's three main points is that science tends to reify its concepts. He also raises the point that facts are not the "written in stone" data we often believe them to be. Rather they are living, breathing, reflections of the times in which we live.)

Keats, John. (1884). *Ode to A Grecian Urn.* from The Poetical Works of John Keats. London: Macmillan.

Appendix

Playing With Words— Finding Your Wise Men

Why Play the Game?

All searches for personal truth begin with learning to see the four wise men. Leave even one of them out and you'll struggle to find your truth. Learn to play their game, however, and your blind spots will be revealed. At which point, you'll be well on your way to finding your personal truth.

You'll also be well prepared for what's coming in Book II—unraveling human nature—and Book III—solving the mysteries of the universe. Not that what's in these two books doesn't stand on it's own. It does. But since the wise men's game lays the foundation for these two books, if you learn to play it, your ability to gain from these books will increase exponentially.

How is this possible? Because what you're about to learn will tell you how much of your mind you're using—and how much lays idle. You'll also learn which truths you value and which you ignore. You may even heal a few wounds, albeit, I can't promise that. But even if this doesn't happen, playing the game will change your life.

Of course, in order to do this, you'll need to learn to interpret these games. With this in mind, I've included a few actual games, some of which healed something in the explorer. Please know that I've chosen these games not because of this healing, but rather because the questions they explore get asked so often.

Constructing the Game

Of course, before you can play, you'll first need to construct the game. You'll find everything you need at your local office-supply store. Buy a sharpie pen, and packages of 3 x 5 cards in each of the following colors—yellow, green, blue, pink, orange and white. Then set aside the orange cards.

Now use white cards to make the four elements of truth cards—the mind, body, real world, and theoretical world cards. These cards define the four wise men's realms. Next, make the four kingdom cards. Here, you'll use a yellow card to represent the materialist wise man's realm and his truth; facts—a green card to represent the empirical wise man's realm and his truth; stories—a blue card to represent the rationalist wise man's realm and his truth; ideas—and a pink card to represent the spiritual wise man's realm and his truth; feelings.

Are you into crafts? Then you might want to photocopy the drawings of the four kingdom cards, then glue them to heavy card stock. This can be helpful, as these drawings include descriptions of the realms. Whatever you do though, please don't get hung up on how you construct the game. Or on getting the colors of the cards right. White cards reveal just as much truth as colored ones. And torn strips of paper work just as well as a set of perfectly crafted cards.

I, myself, use a set of laminated game cards. But I've also, at times, drawn the game layout on a piece of pad paper, then used white 3 x 5 cards for the quest and process cards. You might also give a kindergartner crayons and ask her to draw these cards for you. Or if you're good with your hands, you might craft a set out of an exotic wood.

Whatever you decide, just be sure your game cards reflect you and your personal truth.

Getting Yourself Ready

Once you've constructed the game cards, you'll almost be ready to play. Before you can begin though, you'll first need to remind yourself of your goal. All of us, by nature, tend to favor one wise man and ignore the rest. This keeps us from finding our personal truth. The game can reveal these blind spots in twenty minutes or less. Thus, this simple game can unlock your ability to know yourself.

Also remember, before you can play the game, you must chose a guide. The wise men can be very devious, and this person will need to protect you from them. Choose wisely, then, as your success will in part depend on the skills and focus of your guide. As well as on your ability and willingness to accept this person's help.

Your guide will need to remind herself of her goals as well. She will need to act as compassionate observer, protector of your truth, conservator of the kingdoms, and secretary to your mind. She must be able to silently and without hesitation assign each of your responses to the realm of a wise man. I'll explain how to do this in a moment. Moreover, she must do this with childlike openness, seeing all while judging nothing.

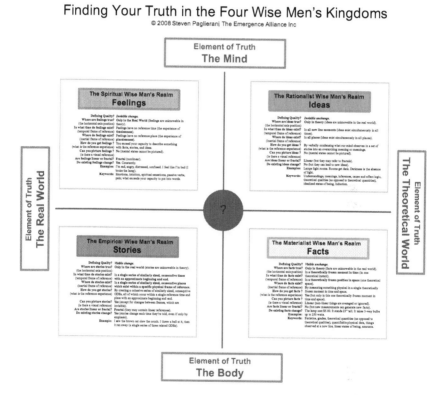

Finding Your Truth in the Four Wise Men's Kingdoms
© 2008 Steven Paglierani The Emergence Alliance Inc

Laying Out the Game and Recalling the Rules

Now clear your mind and relax your body while your guide lays out the game. Know that she should orient the game so that it's facing you. To do this, she should place the materialist wise man's kingdom card nearest to your right hand. She should then lay out the rest of the cards as I have in the drawing I've placed above.

The Spiritual Wise Man's Realm
Feelings

Defining Quality?	*Invisible change.*
Where are feelings true?	**Only in the Real World**
(the horizontal axis position)	(feelings are unknowable in theory).
In what time do feelings exist?	**Feelings have no reference time**
(temporal frame of reference)	(the experience of timelessness).
Where do feelings exist?	**Feelings have no reference place**
(inertial frame of reference)	(the experience of placelessness).
How do you get feelings?	You exceed your capacity to describe something
(what is the reference experience)	with facts, stories, and ideas.
Can you picture feelings?	**No** (mental states cannot be pictured).
(is there a visual reference)	
Are feelings linear or fractal?	**Fractal** (nonlinear).
Do existing feelings change?	**Yes.** Constantly.
Examples:	I'm sad, angry, distressed, confused. I feel like I'm bad (I broke the lamp).
Keywords:	Emotions, intuition, spiritual sensations, passive verbs, pain; what exceeds your capacity to put into words.

The Empirical Wise Man's Realm
Stories

Defining Quality?	*Visible change.*
Where are stories true?	**Only in the real world**
(the horizontal axis position)	(stories are unknowable in theory).
In what time do stories exist?	In a single series of similarly sized, consecutive
(temporal frame of reference)	times with an approximate beginning and end.
Where do stories exist?	In a single series of similarly sized, consecutive
(inertial frame of reference)	places within a specific physical frame of reference.
How do you get stories?	By creating a cohesive series of similarly sized,
(what is the reference experience)	consecutive ODEs in a single reference time and place with an approximate beginning and end.
Can you picture stories?	**Yes** (except for changes between frames, which are
(is there a visual reference)	invisible).
Are stories linear or fractal?	**Fractal** (they may contain linear references).
Do existing stories change?	**Yes** (stories change each time they're told, even if only by emphasis).
Example:	I saw the cat claw the couch. I threw a ball at it, then it ran away (a single series of three related ODEs).

The Rationalist Wise Man's Realm
Ideas

Defining Quality?	*Invisible unchange.*
Where are ideas true?	**Only in theory**
(the horizontal axis position)	(ideas are unknowable in the real world).
In what time do ideas exist?	**In all now line moments**
(temporal frame of reference)	(ideas exist simultaneously in all times).
Where do ideas exist?	**In all places**
(inertial frame of reference)	(ideas exist simultaneously in all places).
How do you get ideas ?	By verbally condensing what your mind observes in
(what is the reference experience)	stories into an overarching meaning or meanings.
Can you picture ideas ?	**No** (mental states cannot be pictured).
(is there a visual reference)	
Are ideas linear or fractal?	**Linear** (but they may refer to fractals).
Do existing ideas change?	**No** (but they can lead to new ideas).
Examples:	Lamps light rooms. Rooms get dark. Darkness is the absence of light.
Keywords:	Understandings, meanings, inferences, cause and effect logic, theoretical qualities (as opposed to quantities), idealized states of being, induction.

The Materialist Wise Man's Realm
Facts

Defining Quality?	*Visible unchange.*
Where are facts true?	**Only in theory**
(the horizontal axis position)	(facts are unknowable in the real world).
In what time do facts exist?	**In a theoretically frozen moment in time**
(temporal frame of reference)	(in one theoretical instant).
Where do facts exist?	**In a theoretically frozen position in space**
(inertial frame of reference)	(one theoretical space).
How do you get facts ?	By measuring something physical in a single
(what is the reference experience)	theoretically frozen moment in time and space.
Can you picture facts ?	**Yes** (but only in this one theoretically frozen
(is there a visual reference)	moment in time and space).
Are facts linear or fractal?	**Linear** (non-linear things are averaged or ignored).
Do existing facts change?	**No** (but new measurements can generate new facts).
Examples:	The lamp cost $5.00. It stands 23" tall. It takes 3-way bulbs up to 250 watts.
Keywords:	Statistics, grades, theoretical quantities (as opposed to qualties), quantifiable physical data, things observed at a now line, linear states of being.

Next, she should place stacks of blank, 3 x 5 process cards—one stack for each color—within her easy reach. She'll be recording your responses on these cards. She should then remind you of the rules, beginning with that you are allowed up to twelve process cards per game. You need not use all twelve. You must use at least four.

She should also remind you that you must answer spontaneously—without hesitation—and without effort. In other words, you must not try to control what you are saying. Thus, while finding personal truth normally requires cards on all four wise men, you must not will this to happen. Rather, for your mind to reveal what you need to know, it must be free.

In addition, she should remind you that there are no wrong answers. Whatever you say, no matter how odd, can lead to your personal truth.

Finally, your guide should reassure you that she will not judge you. Nor pressure you to have an answer.

Now take a few deep breaths.

You are ready to begin the game.

Playing the Game

At this point, your guide should ask you to identify something you wish to explore. Remember, you can choose only one quest per game, and the best quests just pop into your head. Your guide should then record this quest—along with your name and date—on an orange quest card. She should then place this card at the Axis Mundi point.

Now allow this topic to freely float through your mind. Know that whatever comes into your mind—no matter how seemingly trivial and off topic—is a step toward finding your truth. Do your best, then, to honor each thought by speaking it aloud, uncensored and unedited. Then while the guide records your response, silently return to your quest.

Knowing Where to Place the Process Cards

Guides should first mentally assign each response to a wise man's kingdom. Then she should record these thoughts and impressions on an appropriately-colored process card. In addition, in the upper left-hand corners, she should number these cards in the order in which they appear, 1 through 12.

How do you know where to place these cards? The following descriptions may help.

One. If a process card refers to something you can see, then it goes into one of the body's two realms—facts or stories. Both refer to *visible* things. But if a process card refers to something you can't see, then it goes into one of the mind's two realms—feelings or ideas. Both refer to *invisible* things.

Two. If a process card refers to something that is changing, then it goes into one the two real world realms—feelings or stories. If not, then it goes into one of the two theoretical realms—ideas or facts. Neither facts nor ideas change.

Confused? Then try this.

Does what's on this card refer to *visible unchange*? Then this card is the materialist wise man's truth—facts. Facts are things which are frozen in time—snap-shots and freeze-frames of visible people, places, things, and events.

Does what's on this card refer to *visible change*? Then this card is the empirical wise man's truth—stories. Stories are visible sequences of physical things, changes you can picture.

Does what's on this card refer to *invisible unchange*? Then this card is the rationalist wise man's truth—ideas. Ideas are the labels your mind puts on frozen, unchanging categories of stories.

Does what's on this card refer to *invisible change*? Then this card is the spiritual wise man's truth—feelings. Feelings are changes your mind can sense, but cannot see.

Still confused? Then just do your best. Know we'll address these distinctions in depth in Book III. And remember, the game is based on fractals. So it's patterns you're looking for, not perfection.

Guides, please note, when placing these cards, you should place them so the explorer can read them. As you will be likely be sitting opposite this person, these cards will be upside down to you. You should also remember to use a marker which writes both large enough to easily be read by the explorer and small enough to fit the essence of her responses.

Finally, when the response part of the game is done—either because the explorer has used all 12 process cards, or because she has used at least 4 and feels complete—announce that this part of the game is done.

Now you're ready to process what you see.

Interpreting the Results

Your guide should begin this phase of the game by having you count the cards. First count them by kingdom, then by mind versus body, then by real world versus theoretical.

Now notice if there are cards assigned to all four kingdoms. If yes, then try to find what these cards have in common. This commonality will be your personal truth. If no, then without judgment, take a few moments to notice which wise men's truths seem blocked.

Sometimes, seeing no cards in a wise man's realm can cause you to have an emergence. If this happens, the guide should write this aha on a new card and place it on the Axis Mundi. If nothing comes to you, then don't try to force it. Simply try to take in what you see. And if you pay special attention to what is missing, you'll know what has been keeping you from finding your truth.

For example, in chapter two, I mentioned a game I played with my friend John. In it, he searched for his personal truth regarding his deaf son, Aidan. To my surprise, John had cards on all but one wise man—the spiritual wise man. Yet John is a very warm, caring man. He, in fact, had welled up with tears several times during the game. But when I asked him what he thought about having no feelings cards, he replied, "what good would it do to have feelings about this." At which point, I looked at him, and when we connected, he realized he'd found his blind wise man.

Know each explorer's tendencies can vary based on the topics they choose. Overall, though, games should reveal any ongoing personal biases. Perhaps all your cards will end up on theoretical truths. Perhaps they'll all be on real world truths. Perhaps they'll end up mostly on physical truths. Or they may end up mainly on mental truths.

Whatever the outcome, if this outcome seems to contradict what you believe to be your normal truth, then you might want to play a second, or even a third, game.

And if these outcomes still feel wrong to you? Then you might want to leave the game for another day. To be honest, as long as you answer spontaneously, the game doesn't lie. Indeed, if you still feel discomfort, you can be sure you've hit a blind spot. At which point, you've likely identified something which prevents you from finding personal truth.

What else can you learn from the game?

For one thing, you can connect your topic to the patterns you see. For instance, another friend—we'll call her Laura—was having difficulties with a close girlfriend. So when she asked me to help, we played the game. This time, in addition to recording her responses, I had Laura posit answers for her friend as to what she might say was the problem. And when we were done, the underlying problem in the relationship became obvious.

All of Laura's cards were real world cards. All of her friend's cards were theoretical cards. Imagine trying to work out a personal problem without realizing this kind of difference? In effect, Laura was processing this problem personally—as in, through the eyes and heart of the real world wise men. Meanwhile, her friend was processing this problem impersonally—as in, through the measurements and logic of the theoretical wise men. Here, neither person was wrong. They were just arguing apples and oranges. For Laura, the truth was what literally happened—for her friend, what it meant.

Finally, one last thing.

Guides should remember to always respect what comes out of people's minds, no matter how seemingly disconnected or absurd. The mind will always supply exactly what is needed to lead a person to her truth. At the same time, the wise men always pressure explorers to repackage this material—to censor and revise their thoughts and impressions. So if you're the guide, make sure you keep encouraging your explorer to not give in.

Now let's look at a few actual games. Nothing in great detail, just a few examples of games I've guided and interpreted.

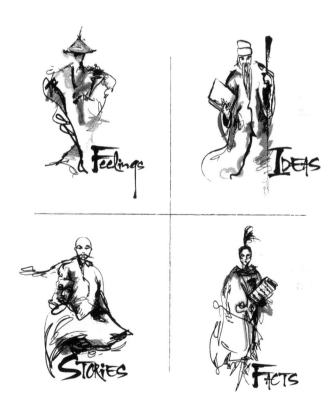

Some Examples of Actual Games

GAME ONE
Quest Card: Am I a hypochondriac?
Process card 1—Probably, but let me tell you why (idea).
Process card 2—I'm five years old in my bathroom. I have a stomach flu. I am scared. My mother is with me (story).
Process card 3—This is the earliest memory I have of being sick and afraid (idea).
Process card 4—I felt scared and afraid to die (idea).
Process card 5—I haven't liked being out of control of my body since then (idea).
Process card 6—She is the only one I feel comfortable talking to about it. My mom (idea).
Process card 7—It's a strange juxtaposition because I am usually a fairly positive person (idea).
Process card 8—Now everyone thinks I just cry wolf (idea).
Process card 9—I feel good right now (feeling, then pleasant surprise).

Card count—0 facts, 1 story, 7 ideas, 1 feeling. Mind—8, body—1, theoretical—7, real world—2. Trusted wise man—the rationalist wise man. Blind wise man—the materialist wise man.

This card count is particularly odd considering this person works in a profession where facts are king—she is a medical professional. Seeing this helped her. She realized her anxiety has not been based on facts. She is also normally a very spiritual person. Except, it seems, when she talks about her anxiety—an obvious nod to that she's been criticized for expressing feelings.

Comments—Some might wonder why process card 4 is not a feelings card. It's simple. To be considered a feeling, the person's body must mirror their words. In other words, their words must be accompanied by visible body-feelings. No visible body-feelings, no feelings card. Hence, the idea card.

Also, while card 2 references a feeling, this feeling comes in the midst of three consecutive ODEs, making it a complex story.

Finally, the quest card asks whether she is a hypochondriac. Yet the second card references a real sickness. Conclusion. Her anxiety is coming from a fear that she will be sick, but be seen as crying wolf. And the pleasant surprise card 9 references reveals she had an aha about this connection.

GAME TWO
Quest Card: Why can't I move forward?
Process card 1—I take no action on my plans (idea).

Process card 2—I know I need, and want, to (idea).

Process card 3—It seems, when I think about these plans, I go blank. I'm frozen (feeling).

Process card 4—I've had a pretty overwhelming few days (feeling).

Process card 5—Thursday, I had to drive my motor home on Storm King mountain (fact).

Process card 6—I get distracted when I have more than one or two items on my to-do list (idea).

Process card 7—It's so frustrating (feeling).

Process card 8—It's so stupid (feeling).

Process card 9—It's not like me (idea).

Process card 10—I guess it is like me (idea, then pleasant surprise).

Process card 11—I associate a lot of fear to the frozen state (idea, then pleasant surprise).

Process card 12—Maybe I distract myself to hide the fear and push it away (idea, then pleasant surprise).

Card count—1 fact, 0 stories, 7 ideas, 4 feelings. Mind—11, body—1, theoretical—8, real world—4. Trusted wise man—the rationalist wise man. Blind wise man—the empirical wise man. This person is a mortgage broker and a schmoozer extraordinaire. He's told me his stories are his main way of making business connections. Yet when it comes to himself, it seems, he can't see the good in stories. Nor in facts. He has no story cards, and only one fact card. This may indicate he was once startled as a boy when telling a story, perhaps when he got his facts wrong.

Comments—This person had played the game previously and knew the significance of missing wise men. Yet he left some out just the same. This indicates an honest game, one which is not being repackaged by logic.

Also, Storm King mountain is extremely steep and winding, and his motor home is huge. Thus, while at first, this entry may seem out of place, in the context of failing to complete to-do lists because he's afraid, it fits perfectly. Indeed, I've repeatedly seen examples of these kinds of dream-like associations—times wherein a person's mind offers up seemingly unrelated material which, in hindsight, contains a metaphoric thread of similarity to the rest. To wit, the picture of driving a huge mobile home up a steep winding mountain sounds a lot like what his to-do lists must feel like to him.

GAME THREE
Quest Card: Why have I been so negative?
Process card 1—My stepfather, Ed, died (fact).
Process card 2—I have been grieving (idea).
Process card 3—I felt I was going backwards (feeling).
Process card 4—I don't have a full-time job (fact).
Process card 5—I don't have a sweetheart (fact).
Process card 6—I've been very upset over things I've thrown away in the past (idea).
Process card 7—Due to Ed's death, I thought I'd have to make a major change (idea).
Process card 8—I thought I was going to lose my hobbies (idea).
Process card 9—I got scared—my physical health was starting to deteriorate (feeling).
Process card 10—When Ed was sick, I prayed for him in the chapel (fact).
Process card 11—I felt like I was going to panic (feeling).
Process card 12—I felt I was becoming an obsolete relic (idea).

Card count—4 facts, 0 stories, 5 ideas, 3 feelings. Mind—8, body—4, theoretical—9, real world—3. Trusted wise man—rationalist wise man. Blind wise man—empirical wise man. Despite there being a good balance between the three wise men present, the missing wise man prevents this person from finding her personal truth about this death.

Comments—In the previous game, the lack of stories resulted in a man's being unable to complete planned tasks. In this game, the lack of stories is impairing this woman's grief work. Here, without stories to ground her grief work, she has no way to feel safe within the grieving process, let alone anticipate she will come out of it alright.

Also, note how her mind offered up seemingly unrelated material which contains a thread of similarity—the loss of a stepfather, the loss of a job, the loss of a sweetheart, the possible loss of hobbies, the loss of physical health. This thread indicates that this person—like many people—has a considerable backlog of unprocessed grief. And that each new loss will likely push all unprocessed previous losses to the surface.

Finally, notice that the last entry—her fear that she is becoming obsolete—ties all her fears of loss back to herself. This shows that this person has a strong connection between herself and her life events. And yes, she appears to be quite self-involved. But sandwiched between two feelings cards is a card which states, she also prayed for her stepfather.

GAME FOUR
Quest Card: Why do I overeat?
Process card 1—I always eat (feeling).
Process card 2—I eat mindlessly a lot of the time (idea).
Process card 3—Trying to find something else to do doesn't help (idea).
Process card 4—Today was a good example. I had donuts in my hand. I saw myself ordering them and tried to stop. I couldn't stop (story).
Process card 5—I wasn't hungry (idea).
Process card 6—I wasn't trying to squelch anything down (idea).
Process card 7—It's almost like I was on autopilot, in a trance (idea).
Process card 8—That's really, really scary—not hopeful (feeling).
Process card 9—I think I'm on my way to gaining back all the weight I lost (idea).
Process card 10—I haven't been to a Weight Watcher's meeting in a few weeks (fact).
Process card 11—I keep forgetting the number of my weight—I don't know the number (feeling).
Process card 12—What do I do with the number (idea)?

Card count—1 fact, 1 story, 7 ideas, 3 feelings. Mind—10, body—2, theoretical—8, real world—4. Trusted wise man—rationalist wise man. Blind wise men—the materialist and empirical wise men. The thing to see here is this woman's lack of visible wise men—there are only two body cards. I see this a lot in people who overeat. She also mentions another thing which points to a lack of trust in the visible wise men—knowing she isn't hungry, but eating anyway. More on this in Book III.

Comments—So if this woman has cards on all four wise men, why doesn't she have a personal truth? As I said in chapter one, you can either have facts or fat, and this woman clearly has a wound about RSS facts. More to the point though, when she eats, she also has several telltale signs of wounds—blankness, loss of control, forgetting, logical impotence.

Also interesting is what she's implied in card 6. She states she wasn't trying to squelch down anything. This points to her having taken as true a widely accepted but totally nonsensical belief that the wise men have propagated—that we overeat to squelch down feelings. Yet here she is, on an idea card, reporting that this was not the case.

In reality, logic is but one of the ways the wise men explain away the blankness which follows a startle. You can't change what you can't see. Thus if you don't notice the significance of startles, then you'll be dependent on others for your truth. See chapters ten (wounds) and thirteen (overeating).

GAME FIVE
Quest card: What happens when you die?
Process card 1—You go to heaven (idea).
Process card 2—As I think about it, I don't know (fact).
Process card 3—I believe I'm going to heaven (idea).
Process card 4—(laughing) Even though I don't believe in God—just heaven (feeling).
Process card 5—I don't know where bad people go (idea).
Process card 6—I connect death with God. It must be my Catholic upbringing (idea).
Process card 7—When I think about death, I think of God (feeling).
Process card 8—I was hiking in Utah with Don. We had a horrible fight. We took off in two directions. I walked a couple of miles. Fifteen minutes later, the sun was gone. I lost the trail. Scared—I prayed to God. Suddenly, I found the trail—two hours back. I believe God led me to the trail. Ever since then, I've felt closer to him (story).
Process card 9—I knew I wasn't going to die (idea).
Process card 10—I was scared (feeling).
Process card 11—I didn't die (fact, then pleasant surprise).

Card count—2 facts, 1 story, 5 ideas, 3 feelings. Mind—8, body—3, theoretical—7, real world—4. This woman's wise men are nicely balanced. Yes, she has only one story. But stories often carry more weight than two and sometimes three facts, ideas, or feelings. And this makes sense, considering that stories must contain at least three facts.

Comments—This woman got startled when she got lost hiking. After that, she blamed God for not rescuing her. The proof she got startled? Despite being able to recant her story, she couldn't personally experience God or anything else that happened to her from the point at which she realized she got lost. The contrast between card 10 and card 11 provoked a healing moment in her, after which, she realized she didn't die.

These kinds of realizations—the kind that have been factually or logically obvious all along, but previously unexperienced—are a common feature in emergences. Yet another evidence for how powerful the wise men can be—and how important it is to have all four.

So is any of what she believes true? For her, it is. Moreover, since no one can actually know the ultimate truth (we're not God), all that matters is that her beliefs improve her life. And this game, clarified her beliefs.

GAME SIX
Quest Card: Am I a good mother?

Process card 1—I feel angry and frustrated a lot (idea).

Process card 2—Yesterday, my son came home. I missed him. He was hyper. We started to plant flowers. He broke a pot. I became very unhappy (story).

Process card 3—I should have known better (idea).

Process card 4—It always ends up a disaster (idea).

Process card 5—I moved so he could go to a better school (idea).

Process card 6—I go to a therapist to understand myself as a mother (idea).

Process card 7—I spend most of my time with my son (idea).

Process card 8—A lot of times I don't enjoy his company (idea).

Process card 9—I feel bad that I don't enjoy his company (feeling).

Process card 10—I try hard to be a good mother (idea).

Process card 11—I don't think I enjoy motherhood as much as I thought I would (idea).

Process card 12—I don't like it when my son plays rough with me (idea).

Card count—0 facts, 1 story, 10 ideas, 1 feeling. Mind—11, body—1, theoretical—10, real world—2. Trusted wise man—rationalist wise man. Blind wise men—all the rest.

Comments—Despite the emotional nature of this woman's quest card, she only had one feeling card. And while a second feeling exists within her story, she clearly doesn't see the spiritual side of this part of her life. To wit, this woman reports on 8 out of her 12 cards that she reacted negatively to her six year old son. Despite this, she also lists things she did for him on 5 of her twelve cards.

She also blames herself for her negative reactions, this despite acknowledging that he's a difficult kid.

Clearly, this woman would benefit from releasing her negative emotions. This might even reduce her guilt. But her lack of trust in the spiritual wise man prevents her from doing this.

Ironically, like many genuinely aspiring-to-be-spiritual people, this woman lives in her head. Yet she engages in many spiritual practices—yoga, meditation, spiritual retreats. And while I'm sure she benefits from these practices, her guilt about being a bad mother—which in reality, isn't even based in truth—prevents her from seeing that she sincerely dedicates herself to her son. Thus she is actually a good mother.

GAME SEVEN
Quest Card: His mohawk?

Process card 1—What does it mean to him (idea)?

Process card 2—Why does he want to draw attention to himself (idea)?

Process card 3—The night I met him in the supermarket, I gave him my number. He asked, "My mohawk doesn't scare you?" I said no (story).

Process card 4—It makes me sad (feeling).

Process card 5—It gives the wrong impression, like he'd rape my daughter (idea).

Process card 6—I'm afraid people will judge him, especially my friends and family (feeling).

Process card 7—It is very out of style (fact).

Process card 8—It looks great on him (idea).

Process card 9—I'm not sure I like it in public (feeling).

Process card 10—I felt safe telling him I have hepatitis C (idea).

Process card 11—I expected him to be needy like I am (idea).

Process card 12—I'm taking advantage of his neediness (feeling).

Card count—1 fact, 1 story, 6 ideas, 4 feelings. Mind—10, body—2, theoretical—7, real world—5. Trusted wise man—rationalist wise man. Blind wise man—materialist wise man. Yet another person with a preference for the invisible wise men.

Comments—As you may have guessed, this woman recently fell in love with this man. No surprise, she has a fairly good balance of three wise men, but is short on facts. Who cares about facts when they fall in love?

The fact is, he has a mohawk, and she is clueless as to how she feels about it. All over the place, obviously. Ambivalent, as well.

Also, several other falling-in-love patterns are obvious here as well—surprise that she likes someone she would normally dislike, neurotic self-examination, fears as to how her friends and family will see him, etc. Even her comment that he looks like the kind of guy who would rape her daughter gets blown off.

Ah, ain't love grand.

GAME EIGHT
Quest Card: Why are Monday mornings bad?
Process card 1—I don't like Mondays—that's a song (idea).

Process card 2—Last week, I asked myself why I don't like Mondays (fact).

Process card 3—I go to karate. I like that. I go to therapy. I like that (feeling).

Process card 4—Am I working when I do those two things (idea)?

Process card 5—They are work (idea).

Process card 6—Usually, the rest of my day is open (idea).

Process card 7—I'm waking up anxious (feeling, then pleasant surprise).

Card count—1 fact, 0 stories, 4 ideas, 2 feelings. Mind—6, body—1, theoretical—5, real world—2. Trusted wise man—the rationalist wise man. Blind wise man—the empirical wise man.

Comments—To begin with, there are only 7 cards. Why? Because this person had an aha on his seventh card. He realized he liked what he did on Mondays, but didn't like what he felt like when he woke up.

This led him to realize that his impression of Mondays wasn't coming from what he did on Mondays, but rather from what he felt as he woke up. This kind of misunderstanding is common in people whose blind wise man is the empirical wise man. Without stories to ground their ideas, these folks conclude things which often aren't based in reality, even when the other three wise men are present.

Know that the anxiety he felt as he woke up on Mondays clearly indicates a wound—and as you'll learn in Book III, chapter ten, the sure sign here is that he is bracing for pain. In effect, he was expecting all Mondays to be bad days, when in truth he enjoyed what he did.

Another thing that indicates a wound is that he saw no way to avoid bad Mondays. He had no choices.

Lastly, while his cards fail to reference any wounding event which might account for his anxiety, nonetheless, his pleasant surprise indicates healing. No one feels pleasant feelings about anxiety except after they heal. Thus while he may never know what caused this wound, this man healed something anyway.

GAME NINE
Quest card: Why is it so hard to pick a question?
Process card 1—I feel pressured when asked to pick anything (feeling).

Process card 2—I can almost hear someone saying that to me (feeling).

Process card 3—My heart beats faster. I panic (idea).

Process card 4—Panic (feeling).

Process card 5—Hurry up or you'll get nothing (idea).

Process card 6—If I don't pick, I'll lose my turn (idea, then pleasant surprise).

Card count—0 facts, 0 stories, 3 ideas, 3 feelings. Mind—6, body—0, theoretical—3, real world—3. Yet another person who does not trust physical wise men. "Ungrounded" would be one way to describe her. "Living in her head" would be another. At the same time, she does have a balanced awareness of her thoughts. Trusted wise men—the rationalist and spiritual wise men. Blind wise men—the empirical and materialist wise men.

Comments—This woman knows how to self-examine. And how to gain from the game. And despite her total lack of physical wise men, she had an aha. She realized that whenever she was asked to pick a question, she'd choke. Moreover, it's easy to see the ghosts of this wounding scene present in her responses. To wit, it's likely she once got wounded when she was too slow to respond and lost something—a turn, perhaps, or a choice of some kind—a meal, a toy, a gift, a game token.

More important, we even know the exact phrase which is causing her to relive this wound—the phrase, "pick something." We know this because, as you'll find out in Book III, "vivid recall of a painful event" is the number one sign of a wound, and she tells us she can almost hear someone saying this phrase to her. She then follows this with a reference to her body's response ("my heart beats faster; I panic"), followed by a spiritual response (panic), and a logical response (the thought going through her head—"hurry up or you'll get nothing.").

At this point, she realizes that her inability to pick things has been coming from a fear of losing a turn. Ironically, this quality is not something present in all, or even in most, decisions. Moreover, it's interesting to see how she's been connecting her quest card—difficulty *picking* questions—to that she has difficulty *answering* a question. Yet another evidence for that wounds create fractal threads of similarity.

GAME TEN
Quest card: What do I really think about my father?
Process card 1—He's hurt me a lot, but I'm trying to learn to forgive him (idea).

Process card 2—I want to forgive him so it doesn't hold me back (idea).

Process card 3—I wish I could have done this earlier, but . . . (idea).

Process card 4—I hope I can have a relationship with my father before he dies (feeling).

Process card 5—He's a good person (idea).

Process card 6—I think I'll always wonder why he did the things he did (idea).

Process card 7—He's 78 (fact).

Process card 8—He lives in NY (fact).

Process card 9—He has five kids, including me (fact).

Process card 10—He never married my mother (feeling).

Card count—3 facts, 0 stories, 5 ideas, 2 feelings. Mind—7, body—3, theoretical—8, real world—2. Trusted wise man—rationalist wise man. Blind wise man—empirical wise man.

Comments—I've heard these kinds of things from people of all ages, especially when a parent is this old. But this person is a teenage boy and his father is 78. Thus the source of his lack of connection to his father is obvious—he has no stories—neither those which would tell him who his father is, nor any in which they are both present.

What's not apparent from these cards is that he is the only child from a second union. Thus all his siblings have a different mother. This may in part be why he has so few stories. He literally witnessed very few life events involving his father.

GAME ELEVEN
Quest Card: Who was my mother?
Process card 1—The caretaker of the whole family (idea).
Process card 2—The giver of unconditional love to everybody (idea).
Process card 3—A very stubborn person at times (idea).
Process card 4—A person who suffered without complaining (idea).
Process card 5—She was a person who gave more than she should have (feeling).
Process card 6—She was naive (idea, then pleasant surprise).

Card count—0 facts, 0 stories, 5 ideas, 1 feeling. Mind—6, body—0, theoretical—5, real world—1. Trusted wise man—rationalist wise man. Blind wise men—the materialist and empirical wise men.

Comments—This woman was in her sixties when she played this game. Moreover, up to this point, she had, for her whole life, idolized her mother to the point that she constantly felt indebted to her. And compelled to make the same self sacrifice for her own family. Indeed, these feelings had continued to haunt her even after her mother's death. But when the game allowed her to see the downside to her mother's compulsive giving, she began doing things for herself.

To wit, after playing this game, she was noticeably more self caring, at times, doing things for herself even when doing so meant others would have to wait or feel left out. After having spent her whole life serving others, this is nothing short of a miracle.

Please note, this woman had sat in my therapy room for several years prior to this game. Thus while this game clearly changed her, she had been building momentum toward these changes for some time.

GAME TWELVE
Quest Card: How can I get thin?
Process card 1—Eat less (idea).
Process card 2—Exercise more (idea).
Process card 3—Eat more fruits and vegetables (idea).
Process card 4—Get more hobbies (idea).
Process card 5—Eat less fat and sugar (idea).
Process card 6—Smoke more (idea).
Process card 7—More water (idea).
Process card 8—Express myself (idea).
Process card 9—By not giving up (idea).
Process card 10—More sex (idea).
Process card 11—Think positive (idea).
Process card 12—Relax more (idea).

Card count—0 facts, 0 stories, 12 ideas, 0 feelings. Mind—12, body—0, theoretical—12, real world—0. Trusted wise man—the rationalist wise man. Blind wise men—all the rest.

Comments—This woman can't have been trying any harder to lose weight. Can you tell? From her game cards alone, we could guess that she's read every book and tried every diet. And failed anyway. Moreover, most of her ideas are good ones. However, without having a personal truth to guide her, they do her no good and she continues to fail.

How do you find this kind of personal truth? We'll explore this in detail in Book III when we talk about how to heal wounds (chapter ten) and how to lose weight (chapter thirteen). And no, I'm not referring to some new diet or exercise plan. I'm referring to a method by which you can formulate your own truth about food, weight, and fitness.

As for what her game reveals, know it represents the classic pattern for an overeater, a mind first person who tries to control her weight through will-powered mental gymnastics. Here, people use logic to override their body's natural state. To wit, while the majority of this woman's cards refer to doing things which, in theory, can and should lead to weight loss, none of them say *how* she is going to do these things. She has no action plan.

She also has no awareness as to what it looks like to be *naturally* thin. For her, then, losing weight is like trying to sketch something she's never seen before. Moreover, while we often use the word "see" to refer to having a logical understanding, in truth, if you want to change something, the word "see" should be taken literally. None of this woman's cards do this.

The point? You can't change what you can't sketch. Including your weight.

GAME THIRTEEN
Quest card: My problems with doing the billing?
Process card 1—The first thing I do is procrastinate (idea).
Process card 2—I feel nervous and anxious (idea).
Process card 3—I listed all the clients (fact).
Process card 4—Part of the billing, I call the fixed billing (idea).
Process card 5—I did that part of the billing on Saturday (fact).
Process card 6—Then I walked away from the rest of it (fact).
Process card 7—On Sunday, I composed a letter about billing (fact).
Process card 8—The letter spoke about changes in how we do business and in the billing process (idea).
Process card 9—I went to Kinkos. I made 40 copies of the letter. I stopped at McD's for a wrap. I picked up my wife's parents. I came home and went back to work (story).
Process card 10—I finished all of it, then breathed a sigh of relief (idea).
Process card 11—I noticed that as I was finishing the billing, I got into a quasi-state of timelessness—I didn't notice how much time had gone by (fact).
Process card 12—I just realized that I felt anxiety before I started, timelessness afterwards, and nothing inbetween (feeling, then pleasant surprise).

Card count—5 facts, 1 story, 5 ideas, 1 feeling. Mind—6, body—6, theoretical—10, real world—2. Trusted wise men—the theoretical wise men. Blind wise men—the real world wise men.

Comments—In this game, we see a number of things which point to this man having a wound. His anxiety indicates he braces for pain, and when he says he's procrastinating, he's blaming himself. Also, his lack of feelings cards until card 12 indicate the sort of detachment which typically follows a startle, another indicator. Moreover, he makes no direct reference to what he's afraid of. He literally can't see what he's so anxious about.

So did playing this game heal anything? His pleasant surprise indicates it did. But what exactly did he heal?

To begin with, he defined a hole in his consciousness, the time after his anxiety and before his feelings of timelessness. This led him to realize that his previous explanation—that he's been procrastinating—can't be true, and that he must have a wound.

As to why saying he procrastinates means he is blaming himself, we'll talk about this idea in detail in Book II, chapter five.

GAME FOURTEEN
Quest Card: Why I feel so sick?
Process card 1—I don't know what's going to come out (idea).

Process card 2—I don't know what to say (idea).

Process card 3—I feel like I want to check out, curl up on the sofa (feeling).

Process card 4—I'm really scared when I lash out at my son (feeling).

Process card 5—I see him startle (idea).

Process card 6—I apologize to him (idea).

Process card 7—I can't stop it. It keeps happening to me (idea).

Process card 8—It's the first instant, when I start yelling, that startles him (idea).

Process card 9—I can't believe this happens (idea).

Process card 10—A few months ago, we were having dinner. My son said something upsetting to me. I can't remember it. I yelled and told him, "you hurt me." I kept following him into his room, screaming and pointing at him. He was cowering (story).

Process card 11—He's six (fact).

Process card 12—I'm torn between he's six and he's playing me (idea, then pleasant surprise).

Card count—1 facts, 1 story, 8 ideas, 2 feelings. Mind—10, body—2, theoretical—9, real world—3. Trusted wise man—the rationalist wise man. Blind wise man—the materialist wise man.

Comments—Although you might not see it from this woman's cards, I know her to be a warm, involved, loving mother. That even warm, loving mothers lose it doesn't surprise me. Amazingly, it seems to surprise most warm, loving mothers.

This said, what is significant about this game is how card 12 defines her problem—her ambivalent feelings that a six year old boy is playing her. This points to a time wherein she likely got startled by this very thing. Perhaps when she was six, a six year old boy suckered her into an embarrassing situation. Whatever the case, it's obvious that when she loses it on her son, she's reliving a wound. And card 12 shows she realized this.

So did she improve after this? Yes. By her own reporting, noticeably so. Indeed, before this game, this topic had come up many times in her therapy, whereas after this game, she ceased to raise this topic. Ironically, she, herself, failed to notice most of this improvement, and this is common. While all emergences provoke immediate changes for the better in people, it often takes time for these changes to be obvious to them.

GAME FIFTEEN-A
Quest Card: When am I going to be happy?

Process card 1—I've never really been happy (feeling).

Process card 2—How do I control my impulses (idea)?

Process card 3—Where's my gratitude (idea)?

Process card 4—Why do I hurt the ones I love (idea)?

Process card 5—Why are my reactions to things different from other people (idea)?

Process card 6—Why am I so defensive (idea)?

Process card 7—What reason do I have to offend people (idea)?

Process card 8—Why do I have mood swings (idea)?

Process card 9—How do I control my mood swings (idea)?

Process card 10—I keep lashing out beyond reason (idea).

Process card 11—The road less traveled is very appealing (idea).

Process card 12—I never really fit in (feeling).

Card count—0 facts, 0 stories, 10 ideas, 2 feelings. Mind—12, body—0, theoretical—10, real world—2. Trusted wise man—rationalist wise man. Blind wise men—the two visible wise men, the materialist wise man and the empirical wise man. He's definitely a head-with-feet.

Comments—When card 12 appeared, I made a decision to continue writing cards. I rarely do this, but I trusted the spiritual wise man. He didn't let me down.

Process card 13—Five years ago, in March, I got a prescription for my depression (fact).

Process card 14—In high school, I was told I'd never be anything but a photographer (fact).

Process card 15—I only wanted to be a photographer (feeling).

Process card 16—Last Monday, my wife asked me to close the garage door. I didn't do it right away. She closed the door. I lashed out at her. Can't you wait a minute (story).

Card count—2 facts, 1 story, 10 ideas, 3 feelings. Mind—13, body—3, theoretical—12, real world—4. Trusted wise man—the rationalist wise man. Blind wise man—the empirical wise man. Now he's a bit better.

Comments—Note that the pattern throughout this extended game was for this man to trust his mind over his body and theoretical truths over real world truths. Seeing this, I again decided to trust the spiritual wise man once more and did something I had never done before—I decided to play a second game.

GAME FIFTEEN-B
Quest card: What makes a good photograph?
Process card 1—It makes you stand there and look at it (feeling).
Process card 2—It contains emotion (feeling).
Process card 3—It reaches you emotionally (feeling).
Process card 4—It impacts you. It makes a lasting impression (feeling).
Process card 5—It's technically correct—It's sharp with colors that are complementary (idea).
Process card 6—It's mounted in a way that augments the image (idea).
Process card 7—The composition is original (idea).
Process card 8—It tells a story (idea)

Card count—0 facts, 0 story, 4 ideas, 4 feelings. Mind—8, body—0, theoretical—4, real world—4. Trusted wise men—the mind's wise men; the rationalist wise man wise and the spiritual man. Blind wise men—the body's wise men; the materialist wise man and the empirical wise man.

Comments—Can you see the difference between the prior game and this one? In the prior game, this man trusted his mind over his body and theoretical truths over real world truths. But in this one, while he continued to trust his mind over his body, his trust of theoretical truths vs real world truths is now perfectly balanced.

What does this reveal?

When talking about his life in general, and especially his relationships with others, he lives in his head and in theory. Not a very good place to have relationships, let alone, to understand people's reactions to him. But when talking about his love of photography, he enters the real world. He's alive. He's himself.

I've met many people who have this same imbalance, mainly brilliant folks whose special interests drive their lives at the expense of their relationships with others. I, myself, certainly fit into this category for much of my life.

Sadly, none of these insights had emerged in this man, this despite his years of sincere efforts to become more personal. Still, as a therapist, this game certainly helped me to more clearly define the nature of this man's difficulties with people. Including that his difficulty had little to do with his efforts and more to do with the dichotomy between his everyday life and his love of photography.

What's Next?

Okay. So you've just finished the beginner's course in finding personal truth. How do you feel? Accomplished? You certainly should. Hopefully, you've remembered to question everything I've said. No one should mistake another person's truths for their own. I also hope this book has awakened more questions in you than it's answered. Moreover, if you've been diligent, you've written these questions down.

Know that Book II will likely answer a lot of these questions, and Book III will hopefully answer the rest, albeit, when I say "answer," I do not mean this literally. I mean that these two books will offer proof for what's in Book I. In doing so, you'll learn practical ways to find your own answers.

For instance, in the next book—Book II—you'll find a series of rather unique personality tests. These tests are based on something I have yet to introduce to you, a new mathematics called *tipping-point-based math.* Administered correctly, these tests can measure real world things with one hundred percent certainty. As opposed to the squirrelly certainties statistically-based tests offer.

What kinds of truths can this math help you find?

Imagine being certain as to why you and your spouse discipline your children differently? Or why you feel attracted to certain types of people and repulsed by others? Or perhaps, you'd like to know why you overreact so badly to certain words. Or maybe, you'd like to know why you get along with some of your family members, but not with others.

Tipping-point-based measurements can tell you all this and more. Truly, they are a powerful tool for finding personal truth.

Interestingly enough, the game I've just introduced you to uses this same math. Which is why it can change people's lives with nothing more than a few 3 x 5 cards. Indeed, were you to put in the time needed to know the wise men on sight—and were you to construct a therapy based solely on this game—you'd probably heal more wounds in a week than most therapies heal in a lifetime.

Finally, realize that integrating what you've read here will likely take the rest of your life. So slow down, enjoy the process, and trust that your mind will always supply whatever you need to heal, grow, learn, and love. Always. All you need do is trust yourself.

Thanks for sharing this part of my journey.

Warmly,
Steven

Printed in Great Britain
by Amazon